IMAGES
of America

LAKE GUNTERSVILLE

ON THE COVER: This photograph was taken during the dedication of the Val Monte Shores resort in Guntersville, Alabama, on May 4, 1958. Several business owners formed the Guntersville Powerboat Racing Association in 1939, the year of the first boat races. In 1952, the local Jaycees assumed sponsorship. Except for the World War II years, the boat races continued on an annual basis until the mid-1980s. (*Advertiser-Gleam.*)

IMAGES
of America

LAKE GUNTERSVILLE

Whitney A. Snow and Barbara J. Snow

ARCADIA
PUBLISHING

ISBN 978-1-4671-2806-3

Published by Arcadia Publishing
Charleston, South Carolina

Printed in the United States of America

Library of Congress Control Number: 2017948462

For all general information, please contact Arcadia Publishing:
Telephone 843-853-2070
Fax 843-853-0044
E-mail sales@arcadiapublishing.com
For customer service and orders:
Toll-Free 1-888-313-2665

Visit us on the Internet at www.arcadiapublishing.com

In memory of Cora Cooley Gross, beloved mother and grandmother

Contents

ACKNOWLEDGMENTS

The authors would like to thank all those who made this project possible. The bulk of photographs came from the *Advertiser-Gleam*, Marshall County Archives, Guntersville Historical Society, Guntersville Museum, and Lake Guntersville State Park. Anthony Campbell (editor of the *Advertiser-Gleam*), Betty Taylor (director of the Marshall County Archives), Larry Smith (Guntersville historian), Julie Patton (director of the Guntersville Museum), Michael Jeffreys (superintendent of Lake Guntersville State Park), Heather McCann (park operations assistant at Lake Guntersville State Park), and Danny Crownover (president of the Etowah Historical Society) have been most helpful.

Many thanks are also extended to the following photograph contributors: Billy Alexander, George Barnett, Margene Black, Mark Bragg (Bragg's Fish Market), Tony Cooley (Cooley's Grocery), Bobbie Curry, Rosemary Darnell, Lindsey Couch Douglas, Mary Yarber Frank, Jo Starnes Goss, Nancy Gilbreath Graham, Dr. Stephen Henderson, Gail Smith Ingrum, David Jones, Milla Kennamer, William E. "Sonny" Lewis, Bubba Martin (Bubba's II), Johnny Simpson, Kimberly Copeland Stewart, and Buddy Taylor. Mike Jones, owner of Mike's Merchandise, generously loaned us vintage photographs. Chad Opdycke, the general manager of Top O' The River, allowed the scanning of many of the photographs displayed throughout the restaurant. He and Kyle Chamblee went to great lengths using an electric screwdriver to remove the frames, and their combined efforts are most appreciated.

Stories, suggestions, and advice were provided by Louella Alves, Dr. Andrew Brown, Sandra Campbell, Martha Black Handschumacher, Sara Harris, Dale and Kathy Hill, Nancy Gross Hill, Betty McGowin Jones, Nancy McAllister, Lynne McCrady, Terri McWhorter, Jean Ann Moon, Valerie Pailloz, Mary Ann Potter, Angel Wisener Rice, Dr. Julian "Pete" Sparks Jr., Fred Taylor, Macey Taylor, Joni Townsend, Jeannie Wallace, T. Wayne Wigley, Dr. Catharine Willis, Carl Wisener, and Cathy Young. Sonny Lewis, Keith Finley, and Larry Smith aided with picture identification and/or reviewed the completed manuscript. Last but not least, special thanks go to Arcadia Publishing title manager Caitrin Cunningham.

INTRODUCTION

Boasting hills, valleys, bluffs, creeks, and a large man-made lake, Guntersville is a picturesque city in North Alabama. It has been the subject of several local histories, including *The History of Marshall County, Alabama*, by Katherine Duncan and Larry Smith; *Guntersville Remembered* by Larry Smith; *A River Town's Fight for Life* by Julian "Pete" Sparks Jr.; *Celebrating Guntersville: Heart of the Old South; Best of the New South* by the Guntersville Heritage Committee; and *Mississippi Bill and the Indomitable Little Boat* by Robert H. Crumby. Many such works focus extensively on its 19th-century history, especially as it relates to the Trail of Tears, the Civil War, and local personalities. The arrival of the Tennessee Valley Authority and consequent creation of Lake Guntersville in 1939, however, forever changed the appearance, culture, and economy of the city. It is this transformation, one from sleepy cotton mill town to tourist resort embracing the titles "Playground of the South," "Beautiful Lake City," and "The South's Most Beautiful Lake," that this work will explore.

The arrival of the Tennessee Valley Authority received mixed reactions from Guntersville locals. Many looked forward to job opportunities, flood control, and rural electrification, while others feared the confiscation of their land. In the end, the dam was completed in 1939, and on January 16, its gates were closed and the lake began to form. In a little over 10 days, Guntersville had a lake spanning over 66,000 acres. Little did locals realize just how much Lake Guntersville would impact the fate of their city.

Excitement developed in Guntersville with the decision of a group of local businessmen, including Rip Barnett, Lee Matthews, and John Davis, to host hydroplane boat races. In August 1939, the town marveled and reeled at the approximately 50,000–60,000 people who arrived to see the races. There was an obvious shortage of water fountains and bathroom facilities. Homemakers rushed to their kitchens to make lemonade and provide water to the overwhelming number of visitors. With limited hotel accommodations available, locals even rented out rooms in their homes. Some in the crowd resorted to camping or staying on their boats. Travel was so limiting that many were caught in Guntersville's first traffic jam. In 1952, the local chapter of the Jaycees took over planning for the annual boat races, which were held until the mid-1980s.

In 1946, a beauty pageant became part of the Guntersville boat races. Local business owners sponsored young ladies from the community to participate. Contestants were urged to enter the contest to support and bolster civic pride. That year, the swimsuit part of the competition had to be cancelled when a sudden rainstorm forced the contestants to rush home to reset their hair for the evening gown portion of the pageant. Ida Will Willis, the first Miss Guntersville Lake, reigned the following day at the races. She later reported, "It was my first and last beauty contest." Miss Guntersville Lake later became a stepping stone to Miss Alabama and Miss Sun Fun. The beauty pageant succeeded until the late 1980s, when it ended for lack of participation.

A mecca for fishermen, Lake Guntersville is often part of the Bassmaster tour. In 1976, Harold Sharp, tournament director of Bass Anglers' Sportsman's Society, chose Guntersville as the site for the Bassmaster Classic. With the 25 bass fishermen also came editors and writers from newspapers and magazines that focused on outdoor living. Each fisherman was paired with two writers to allow a firsthand view of the tournament. David Long of the chamber of commerce remarked, "This ought to be worth a million dollars in publicity." Locals hoped that the media would promote Lake Guntersville and Lake Guntersville State Park to help attract more visitors to the region. Fortunately, the stunning, mountainous lake country has developed a reputation for boating, camping, and fishing.

Little Mountain State Park was formed in 1947. As early as 1969, plans were under way to change the name to Lake Guntersville State Park, a transition intended to associate the park with Guntersville. In 1974, the Lake Guntersville State Lodge and Convention Center opened. At the time, it had 100 bedrooms and 18 chalets. By 1979, sixteen lakeside cottages, a campground, a 1,700-foot beach, and a tennis court had been added. Over the years, improvement included more walking trails and a beautiful golf course. Today, this park is one of the most visited destinations in the Guntersville area. Guntersville also benefits from its proximity to two other Marshall County state parks: Buck's Pocket State Park (day use only) and Cathedral Caverns State Park.

Over the decades, Guntersville had a number of movie theaters, including the Alamo, the Bonita, the Palace, the Ritz, the Marshall County Drive-In, and the Lake. Bill Harris, the manager of the Lake Theatre, was extraordinarily active in promoting Guntersville. Harris advertised attractions with billboards plus a loud sound system he pulled behind his car. Promotions included beauty pageants, special prices like 25¢ and 50¢ deals, a free movie for children at Christmas, live performances, and of course, concessions like candy, popcorn, and soda.

A favorite of state politicians, Guntersville attracted campaigners like John Patterson, George Wallace, Lurleen Wallace, and both Jim Folsoms. In fact, Gov. "Big Jim" Folsom and his family spent summers and vacations at a cabin on Lake Guntersville. Although a small town, Guntersville was often visited by celebrities, among whom were Lash LaRue, Constance Carpenter, Buford Pusser, Martha Carson, Roy Acuff, Tim Holt, and Percy Sledge. Although myriad notables performed in Guntersville, two of the most memorable were Jerry Lee Lewis and Ricky Nelson. To prepare for Lewis's appearance, Lake Theatre manager Bill Harris rented a grand piano. Due to Lewis's gusto, the piano was damaged so severely that the vendor refused to rent any more pianos to Harris. Nelson's last appearance prior to his death in a plane crash was at Pat Upton's club in Guntersville. Some stars like Robert Mitchum, Louise Fletcher, Gary Burghoff, and Jeff Cook admired Guntersville for other reasons, like its peaceful demeanor, their anonymity, and of course, the lake. Mitchum enjoyed downplaying his fame and coming to the lake to fish. Academy Award–winning actress Fletcher visited in her youth and has a family connection to Guntersville, as she is the granddaughter of the late Rev. J.D. Fletcher. In 2007, Burghoff came to advertise a new recreational vehicle park and said, "Guntersville has a real strong draw, not just to sportsmen, but people, people who want to get out of the big city. It also represents Alabama in a very sunny, nice light. It is a lovely area with the mountains, the lake, the Tennessee River, and, I guess, most importantly, the honesty and friendliness of the people. It is just great here." Cook, of the band Alabama, has a home in Guntersville and, for 10 years, was the focus of a local celebration titled "Jeff Cook Day."

Today, Guntersville's reputation is so intertwined with water that few locals can fathom a time before the lake. Lake Guntersville continues to make headlines, especially in fishing magazines like *Bassmaster. Southern Living* listed Lake Guntersville in an article titled "The South's Greatest Lakes." Local excitement abounds over the fact that in 2018, the hydroplane races that once did so much to spread Guntersville's fame are returning. Given larger lake cities, Guntersville's claim of "Playground of the South" might be deemed presumptuous, but locals see it as that and more. Thousands of tourists also think of Guntersville as the ideal vacation spot, and each year, they descend from across the nation and the globe. In the future, there is little doubt that Guntersville will remain a much-loved tourist resort.

One

The Lake

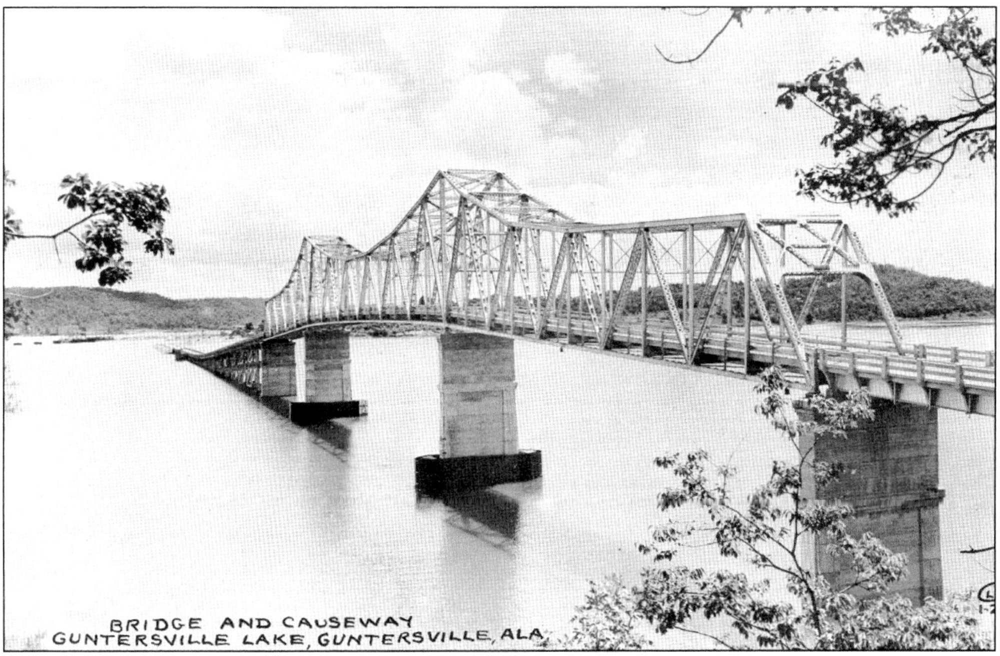

The George Houston Bridge in Guntersville was 767 feet of structural steel and rose 58 feet above water. The bridge was raised 17 feet from its original height to allow for the lake. The depth under the bridge was 50 feet. The two-lane highway across the bridge was considered a marvel in its day. The bridge was replaced in 1992. (Marshall County Archives.)

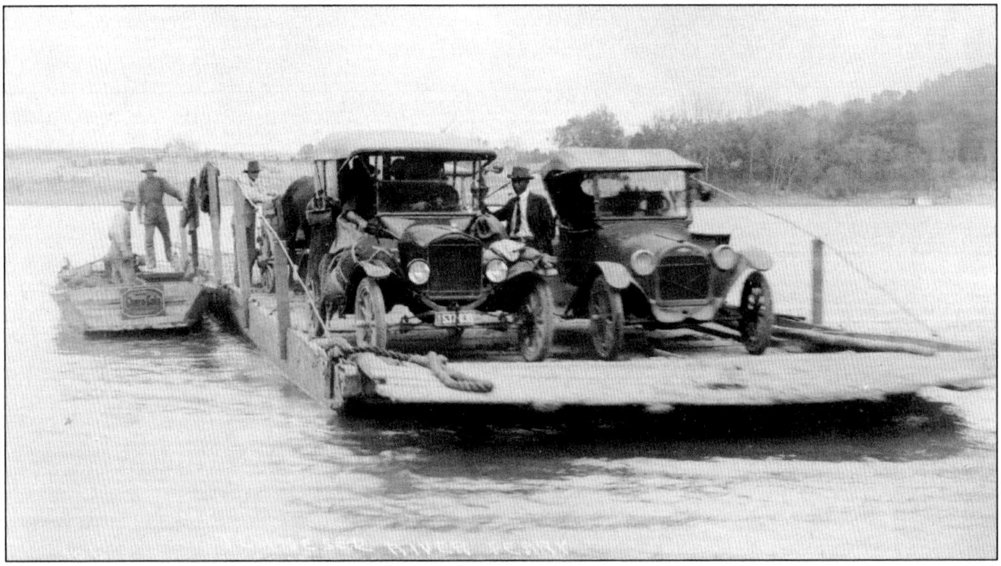

Before the George Houston Bridge, a ferry was used to cross the river at Guntersville. Henry Harrison McGehee operated the ferry from 1923 to 1928. The men in the small boat are Hulett McGehee (left) and Wheeler Walls. Standing at the back of the ferry is Champ Woods. In the front is an unidentified tourist. (Marshall County Archives.)

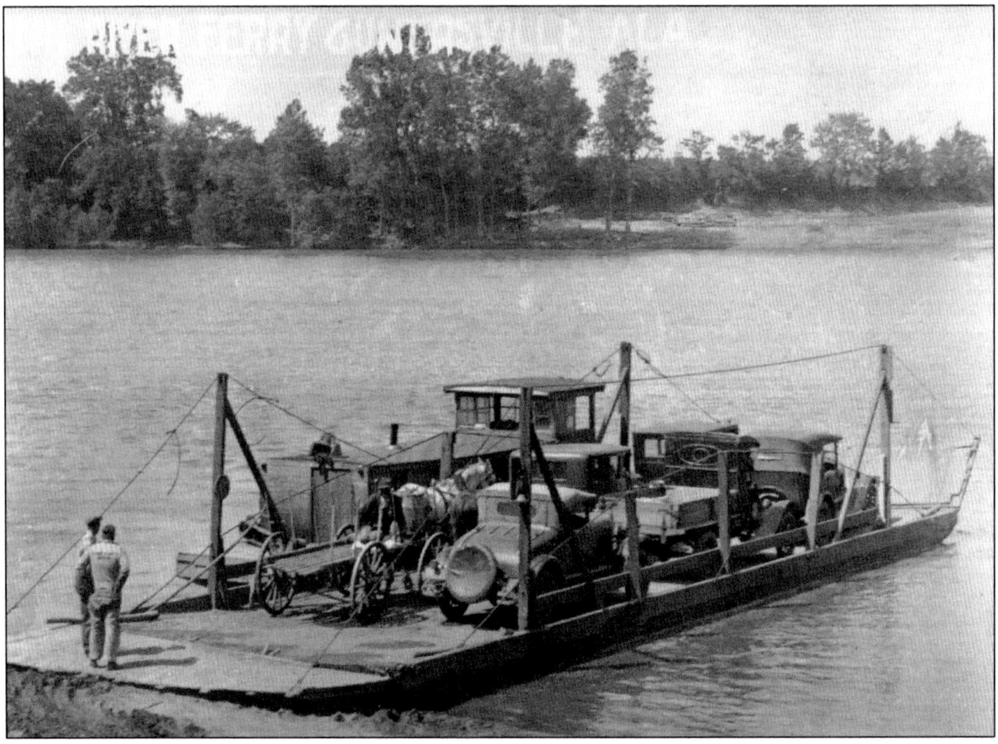

Howard Powell Sr. bought the ferry in 1928, but when the toll bridge opened in 1930, his contract with the county was not renewed. Although the county offered waivers to its residents, the bridge's toll of 50¢ per car plus 5¢ per passenger led Powell to reopen the ferry. (Guntersville Historical Society.)

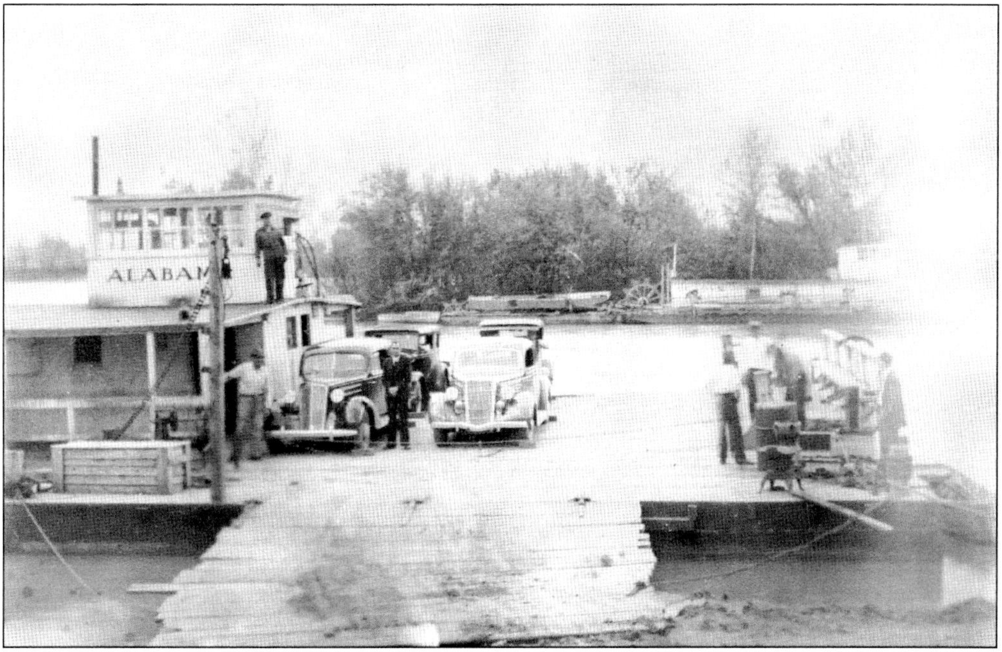

Howard Powell Sr. closed the ferry when the State of Alabama eliminated the toll from the George Houston Bridge. The paddle wheeler *Alabama* is seen in this undated photograph along with Powell's *Gladys* in the background. Powell owned and operated several tugboats and other marine craft as well as a sand and gravel business for roughly 40 years. (Larry Smith.)

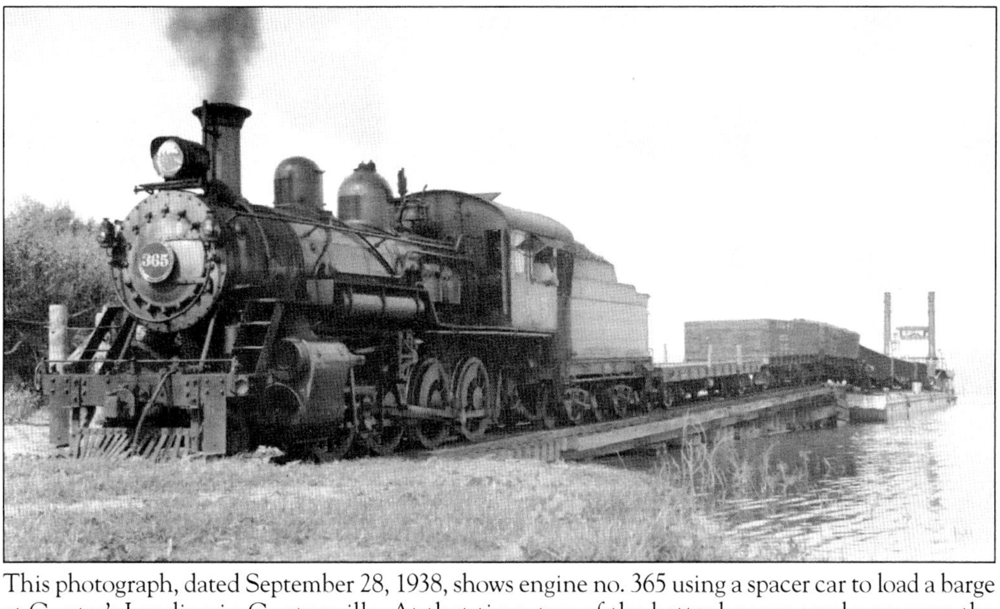

This photograph, dated September 28, 1938, shows engine no. 365 using a spacer car to load a barge at Gunter's Landing in Guntersville. At that time, two of the better-known employers were the Saratoga Victory Mills and the Woodenware Basket Company. At one point much earlier in the 20th century, Guntersville had boasted a Coca-Cola plant. (Guntersville Historical Society.)

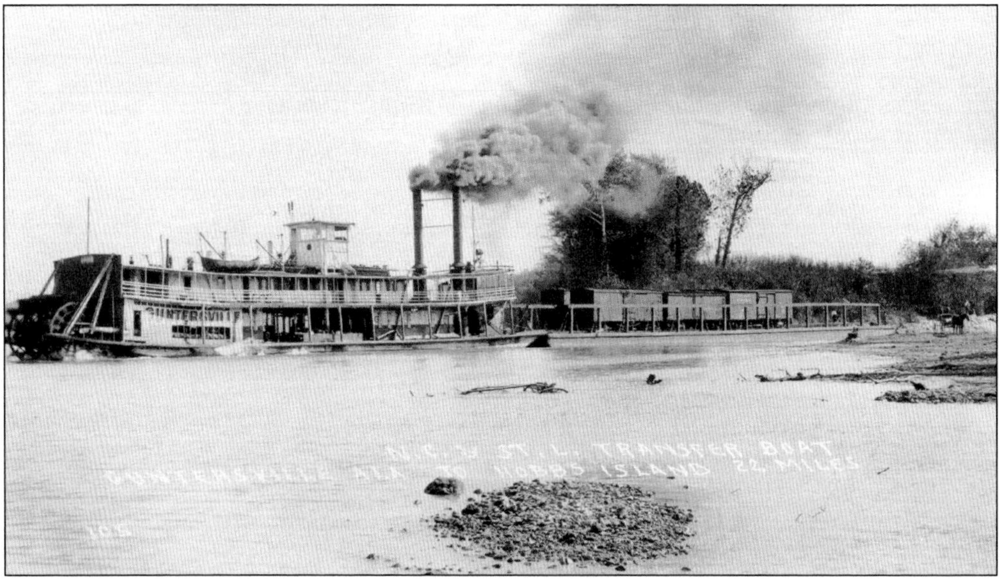

In the early 20th century, the railroad track only went from Chattanooga to Hobbs Island near Huntsville. It was called the Lookout Mountain Route. Specially fitted steamboats connected the breach prior to the completion of the rail system. This image shows a Nashville, Chattanooga & St. Louis Railway transfer boat preparing to move railroad cars 22 miles from Hobbs Island to Guntersville. (Dr. Stephen Henderson.)

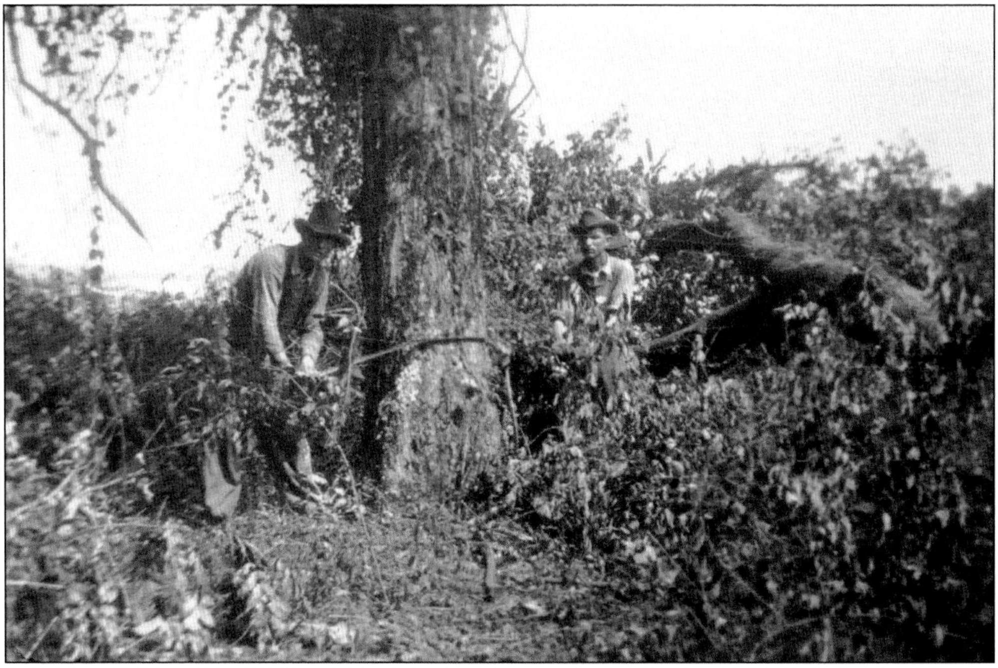

These unidentified workers are helping clear in preparation for the creation of Lake Guntersville. Men were hired to collect brush, cut trees, burn buildings, and move telephone and telegraph lines. Many of the trees were hundreds of years old, so removing them was a tall order. Using basic tools like axes and crosscut saws, the men used teamwork to accomplish this difficult task. (Dr. Stephen Henderson.)

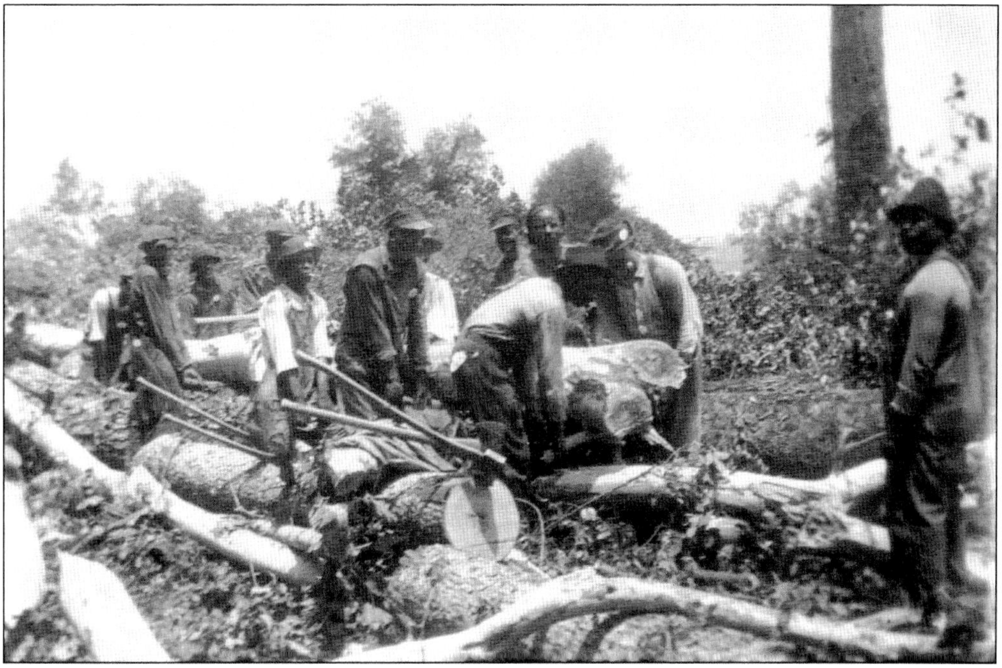

These unidentified workers are also cutting brush to ready for the flooding of the lake. The Tennessee Valley Authority was only one of the New Deal programs to benefit Guntersville. In 1935, under the rehabilitation program of the Resettlement Administration, 100 Guntersville families were impacted. In 1937, a Civilian Conservation Corps project planted one million trees around the Guntersville Reservoir. (Dr. Stephen Henderson.)

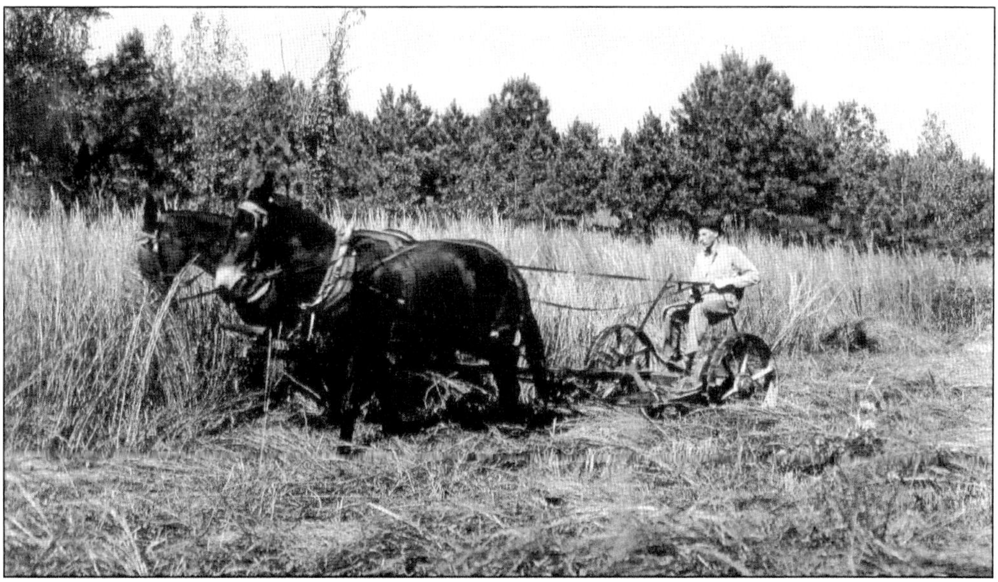

This unidentified man is clearing in preparation for the creation of the lake. Construction on the Tennessee Valley Authority Guntersville Dam began in 1935 but was not completed until 1939. The structure measured 4,000 feet long with gates 40 feet wide. The resulting lake spanned 66,000 acres, quite an increase from the 12,000 acres that had made up the original riverbed. (Marshall County Archives.)

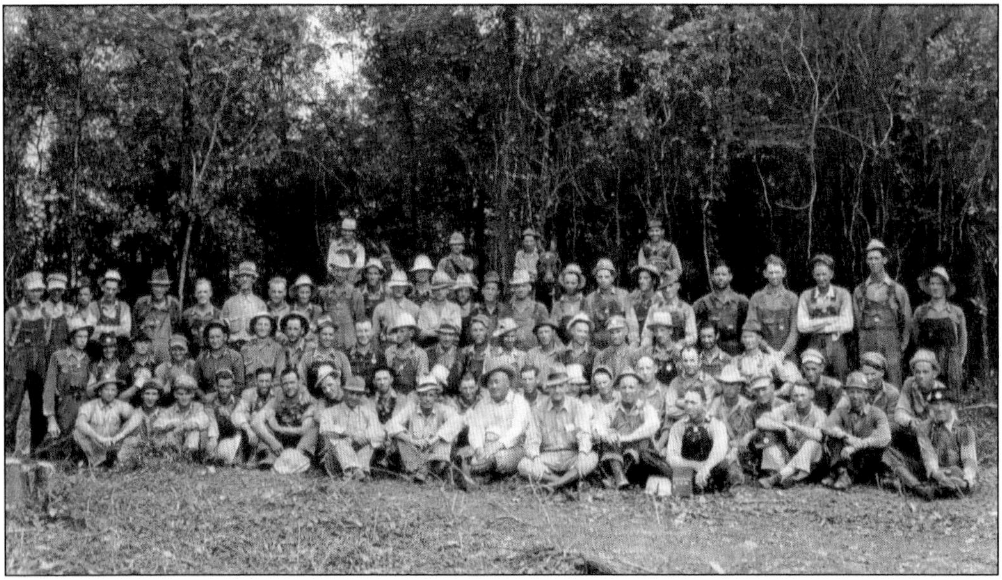

These are unidentified workers at the Tennessee Valley Authority Guntersville Dam. Countless area residents were dramatically affected, as men and boys who had always lived on family farms gravitated to such New Deal projects in the quest for higher income. The opportunities afforded locals enhanced the already popular attitude toward Pres. Franklin D. Roosevelt. (Marshall County Archives.)

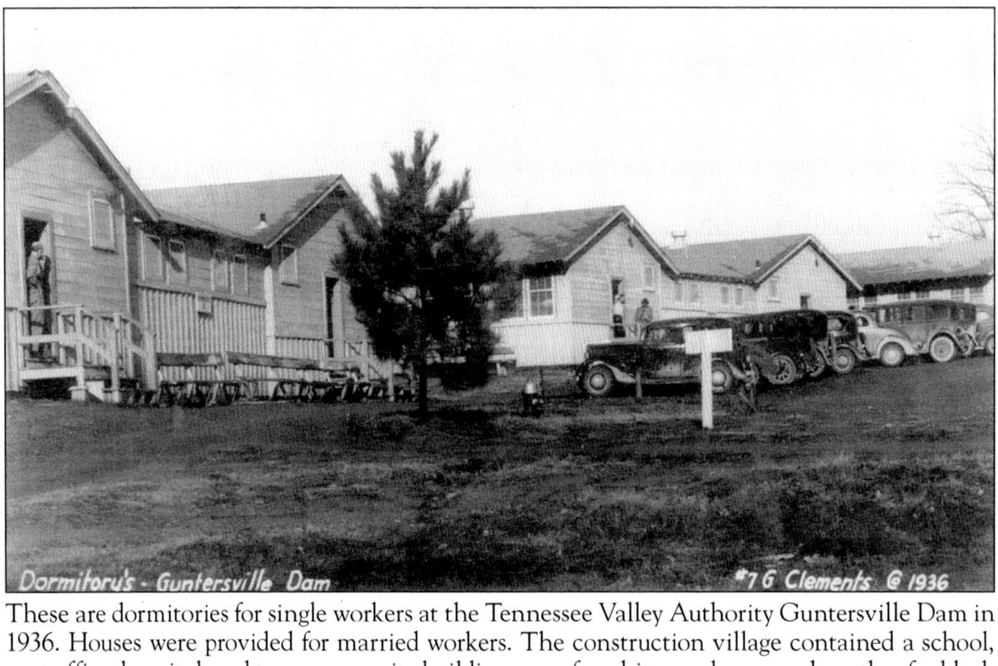

These are dormitories for single workers at the Tennessee Valley Authority Guntersville Dam in 1936. Houses were provided for married workers. The construction village contained a school, post office, hospital, and two community buildings, one for white employees and another for black employees. The dorms and houses were segregated. (Guntersville Historical Society.)

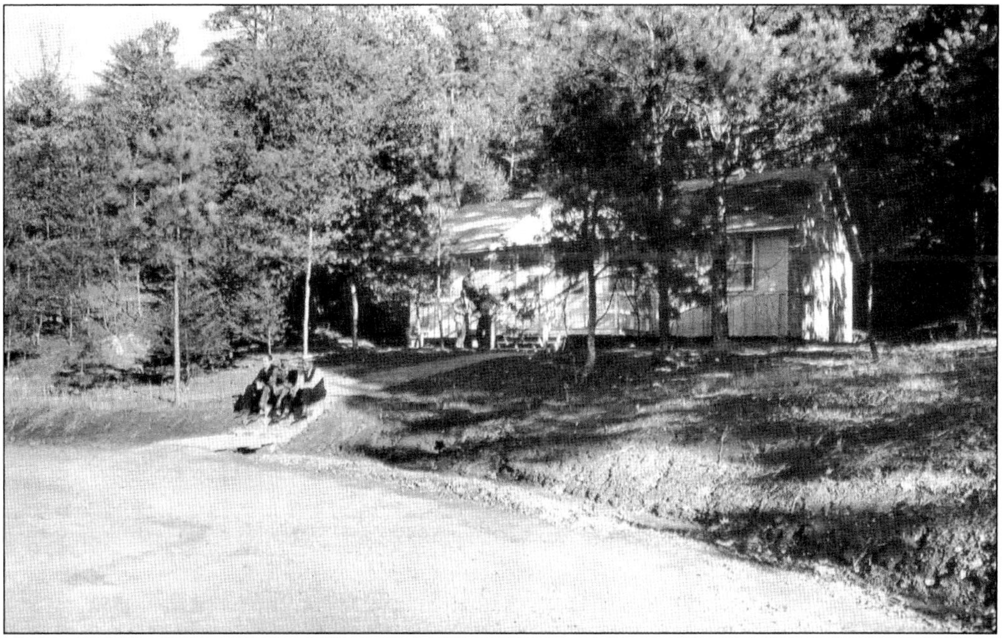

This is the African American community center at the work site of the Tennessee Valley Authority Guntersville Dam. Four unidentified men are sitting in front of the building, while three other unidentified men are shown near the porch. The arrival of the Tennessee Valley Authority shaped lives, regardless of race, and provided opportunities never imagined. (Marshall County Archives.)

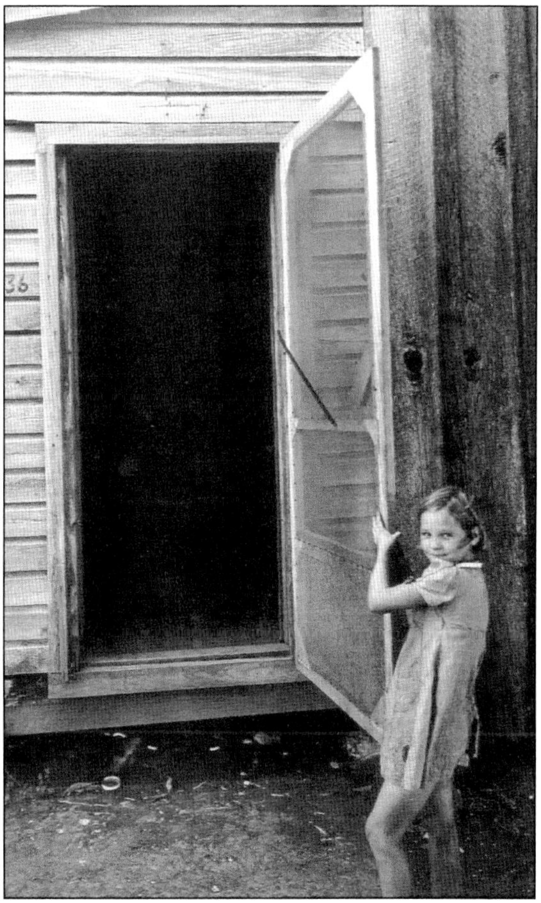

Pictured is an unidentified girl showing a screen door in 1939. The Wheeler Reservoir Screening and Proofing Project attempted to reduce mosquitos and control malaria in the region. The Tennessee Valley Authority had work crews add wire screens in addition to floor, wall, and chimney coverings to residents' homes to ameliorate the spread of malaria and improve the area's quality of life. (Marshall County Archives.)

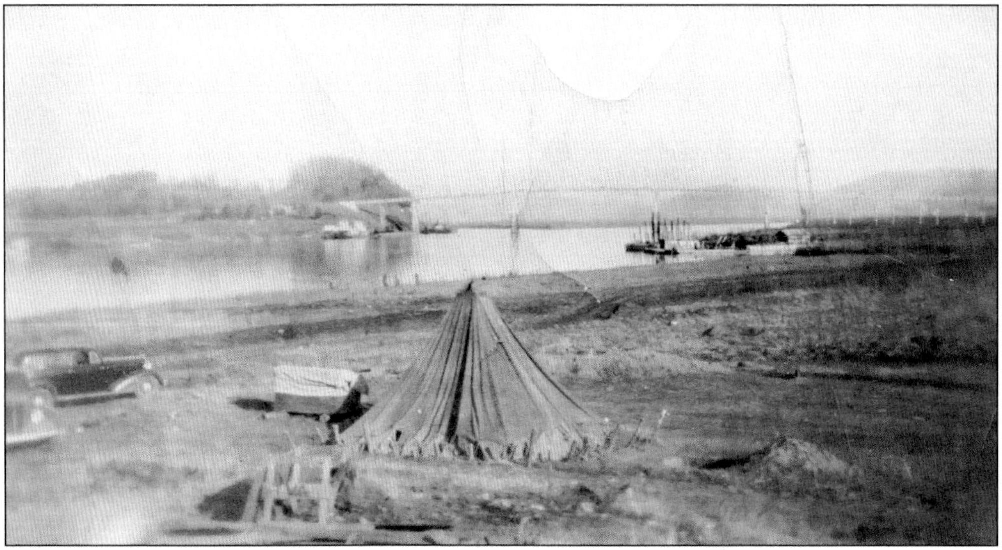

This image of an archeological camp was taken the Sunday before the formation of Lake Guntersville. The photographer was standing atop an Indian mound. That same day, Jess Duncan and Mary Lusk stood atop the mound and posed for a snapshot. Bulldozers partially destroyed the pyramid-type structure prior to the flooding. (Gail Smith Ingrum.)

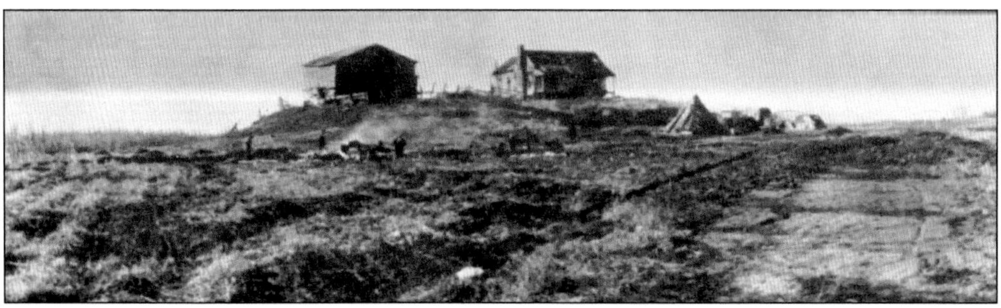

This is the aforementioned Indian mound the Sunday before the water rose to create the lake in 1939. The Tennessee Valley Authority decided to flatten it so as to protect potential boat traffic and barges. Today, the mound's remnant can still be discerned with a depth finder, and it appears as a large truncated pyramid. (Larry Smith.)

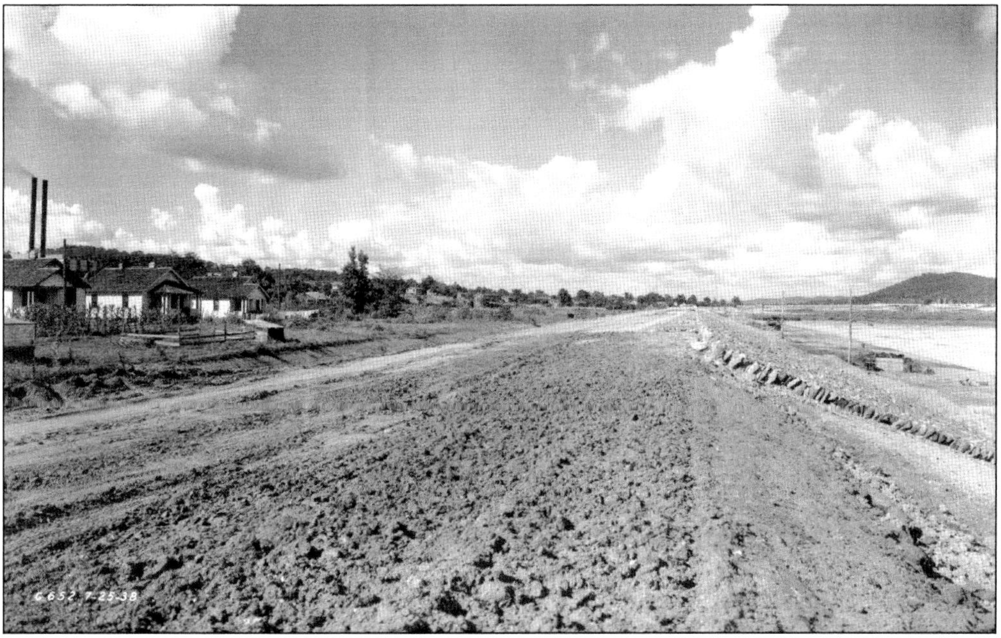

Taken on July 25, 1938, this image shows construction of the levee near the Saratoga Victory Mills in Guntersville. Besides this levee, a water filtration and sewage station was built in preparation for Lake Guntersville. The first managers of the latter were Cleo Manning and Glen Norrell. (Guntersville Historical Society.)

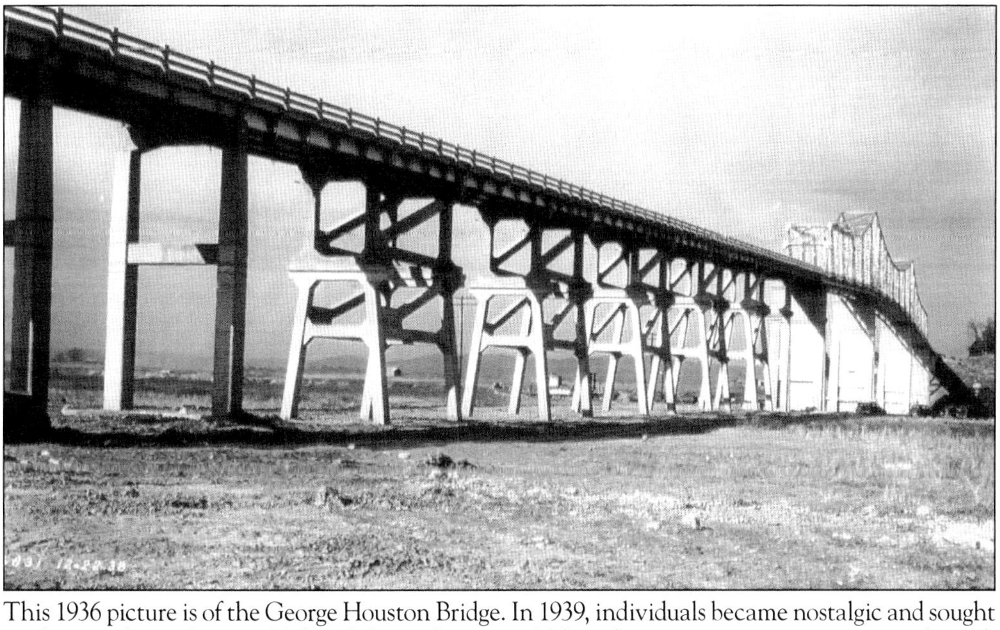

This 1936 picture is of the George Houston Bridge. In 1939, individuals became nostalgic and sought to glimpse places that would shortly be underwater. Although many cemeteries were transplanted, time restraints prevented complete removal. Some Native American artifacts were salvaged, but not all digs were explored. According to Dr. Andrew Brown, "As the water was rising, we were inundated with raccoons, snakes, and gophers." (Marshall County Archives.)

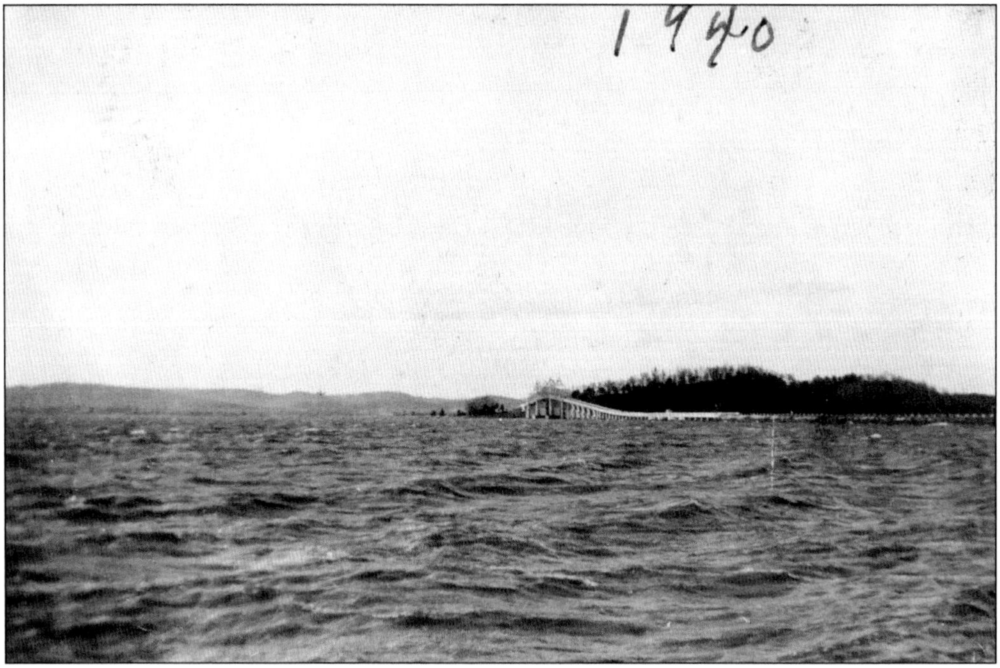

This image, taken in 1940, shows the new Lake Guntersville. It took 11 days for the lake to appear after the Tennessee Valley Authority Guntersville Dam closed its gates on January 16, 1939. Though many locals saw it as a new beginning for the city, others, especially those who watched their farms disappear, were devastated. (Marshall County Archives.)

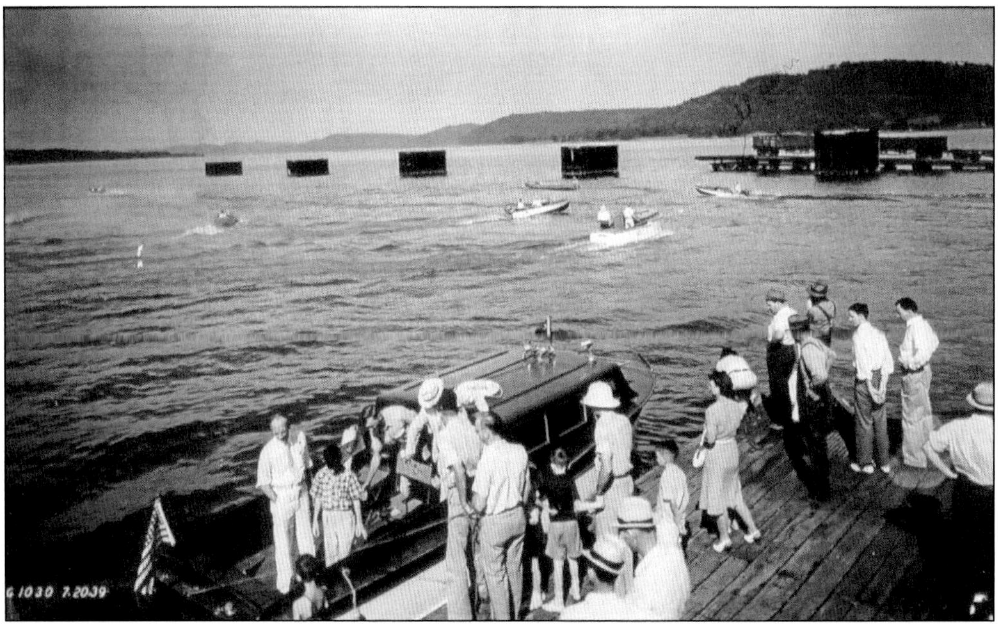

Pictured is the Guntersville Harbor on July 20, 1939. The boat near the dock belonged to Gus King, who provided boat rides to excited individuals of all ages. Among the men in the photograph are Bill Prickett and Lester Johnson. In the far-right background is Bill Harris driving a boat. (Marshall County Archives.)

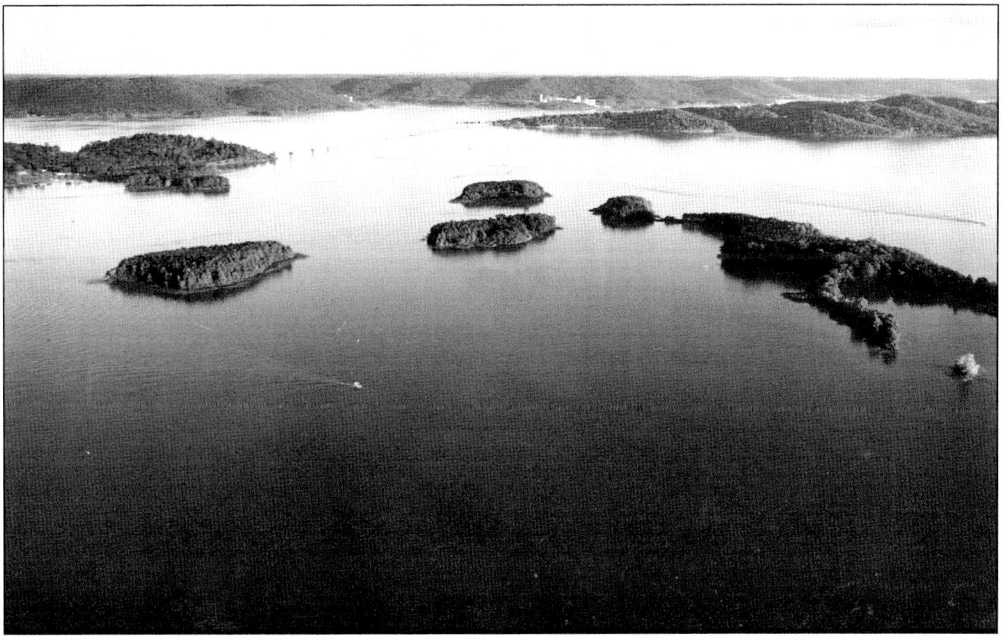

Scattered islands dot Lake Guntersville. Today, many trees on some of the islands are bare because of cormorant droppings. The islands, especially Goat Island, are popular places to fish for bream, bass, and catfish. Throughout the post-lake decades, stories of couples and hermits living on the islands occasionally appeared in the local newspaper. (*Advertiser-Gleam.*)

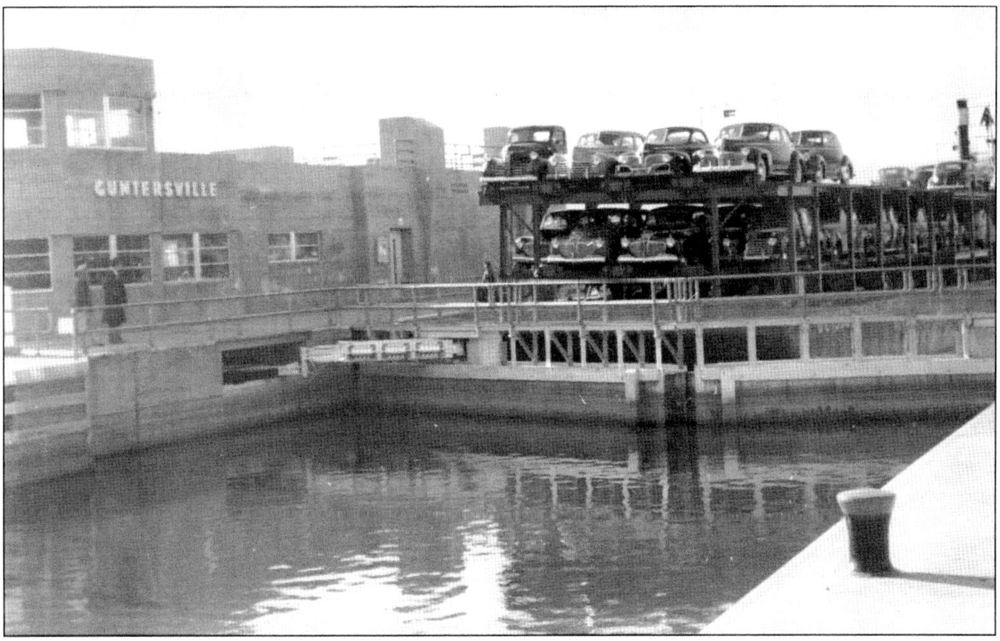

This barge, owned by Commercial Carriers in Guntersville's Northtown, is transporting automobiles by locking through the Tennessee Valley Authority Guntersville Dam in 1941. Commercial Carriers employed many locals. When cranes were not used, local teens earned 12¢ per car to drive the cars off the barge. From Guntersville, the automobiles, mostly Dodges, Plymouths, and Chryslers, were transported by truck. (Guntersville Historical Society.)

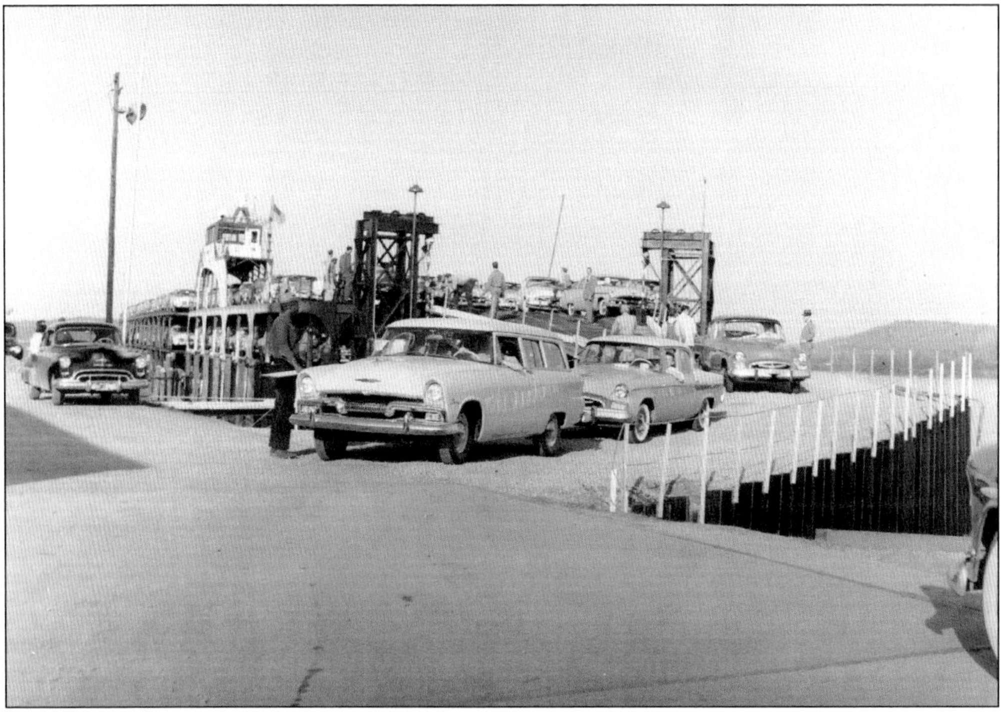

The original location of Commercial Carriers was a concrete dock at the foot of Scott Street. After World War II, its business location was moved to the end of Worth Street. When Commercial Carriers transferred them from the river barges to trucks, the cars brought sightseers and gawkers. (Guntersville Historical Society.)

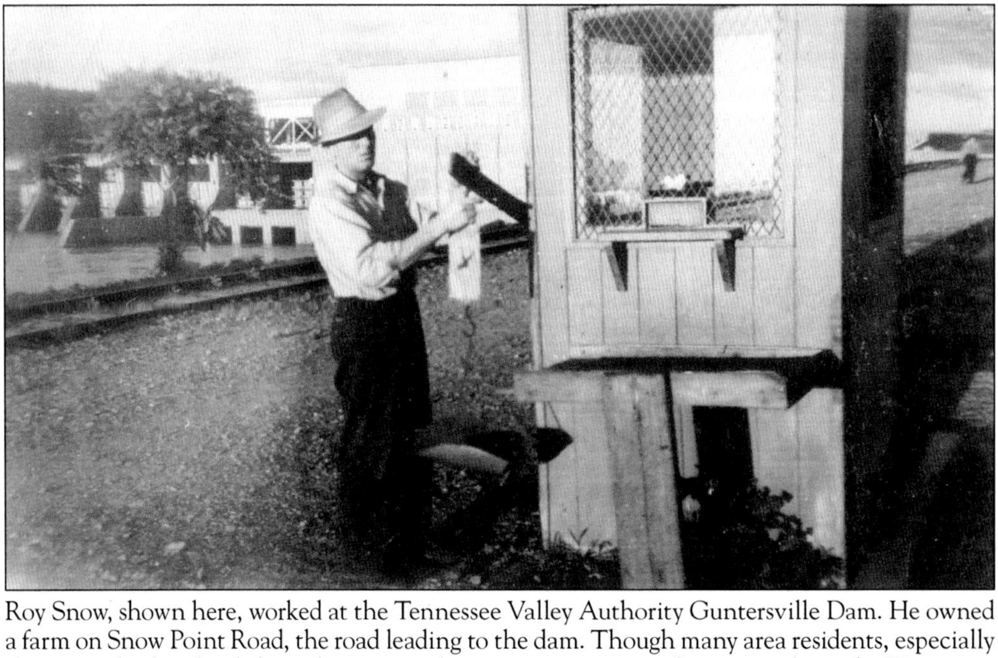

Roy Snow, shown here, worked at the Tennessee Valley Authority Guntersville Dam. He owned a farm on Snow Point Road, the road leading to the dam. Though many area residents, especially the ones who lost land through eminent domain, were unsure of or angry about the Tennessee Valley Authority, others like Roy saw it as an employment opportunity. (Authors' collection.)

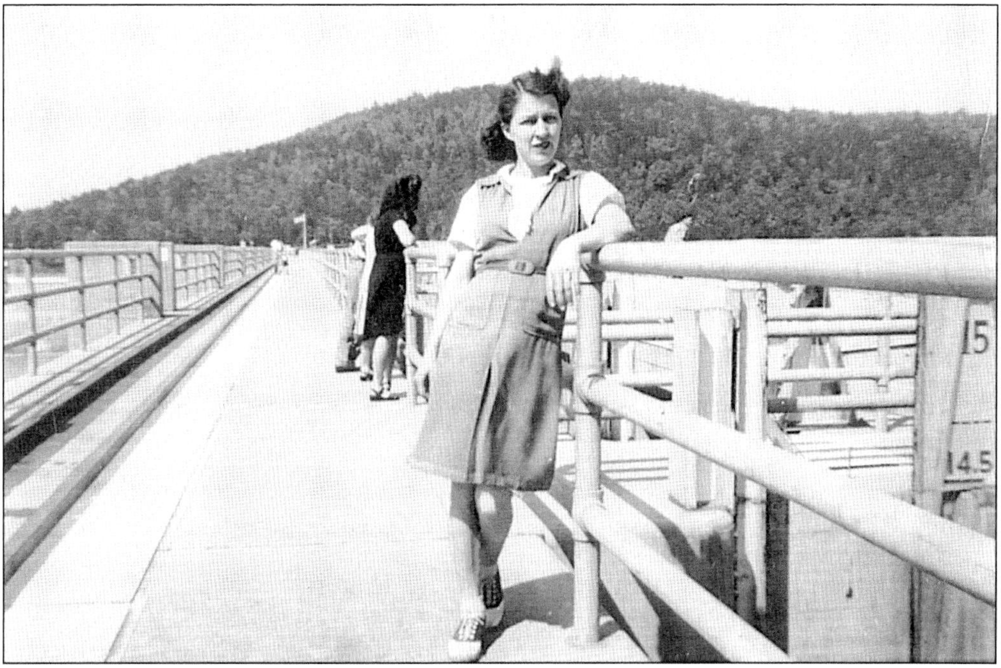

Gladys Snow, wife of Roy Snow, is shown standing on the crosswalk above the Tennessee Valley Authority Guntersville Dam. This crosswalk allowed visitors to walk from one side of the river to the other. From this perch, they could look inside the various gates to see turtles, fish, and floating debris, plus activities in the locks. Because of security concerns, this walkway was closed after 9/11. (Authors' collection.)

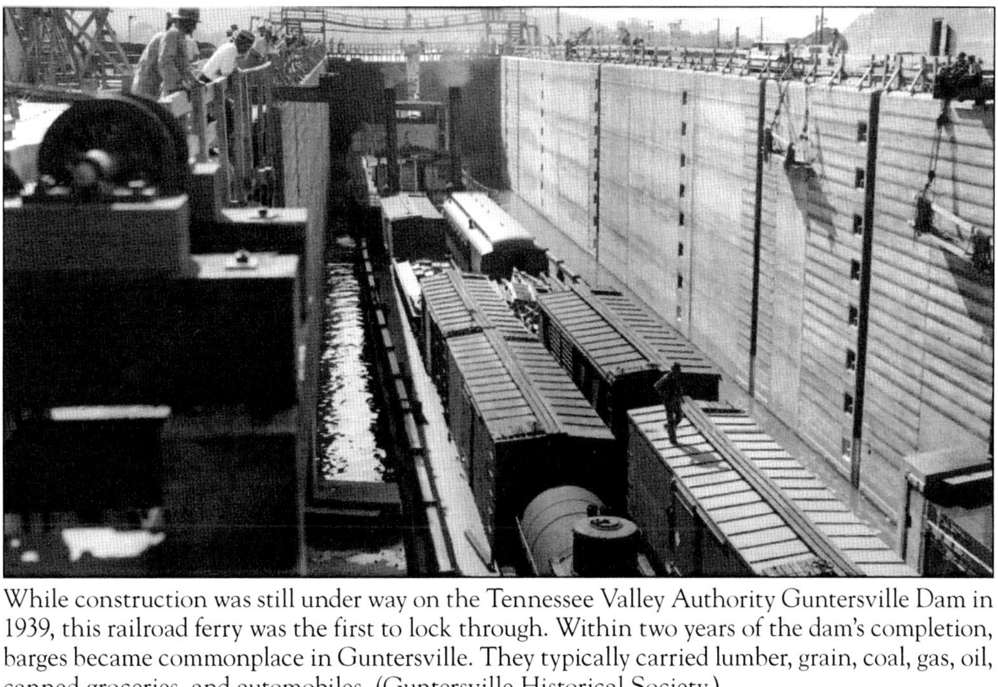

While construction was still under way on the Tennessee Valley Authority Guntersville Dam in 1939, this railroad ferry was the first to lock through. Within two years of the dam's completion, barges became commonplace in Guntersville. They typically carried lumber, grain, coal, gas, oil, canned groceries, and automobiles. (Guntersville Historical Society.)

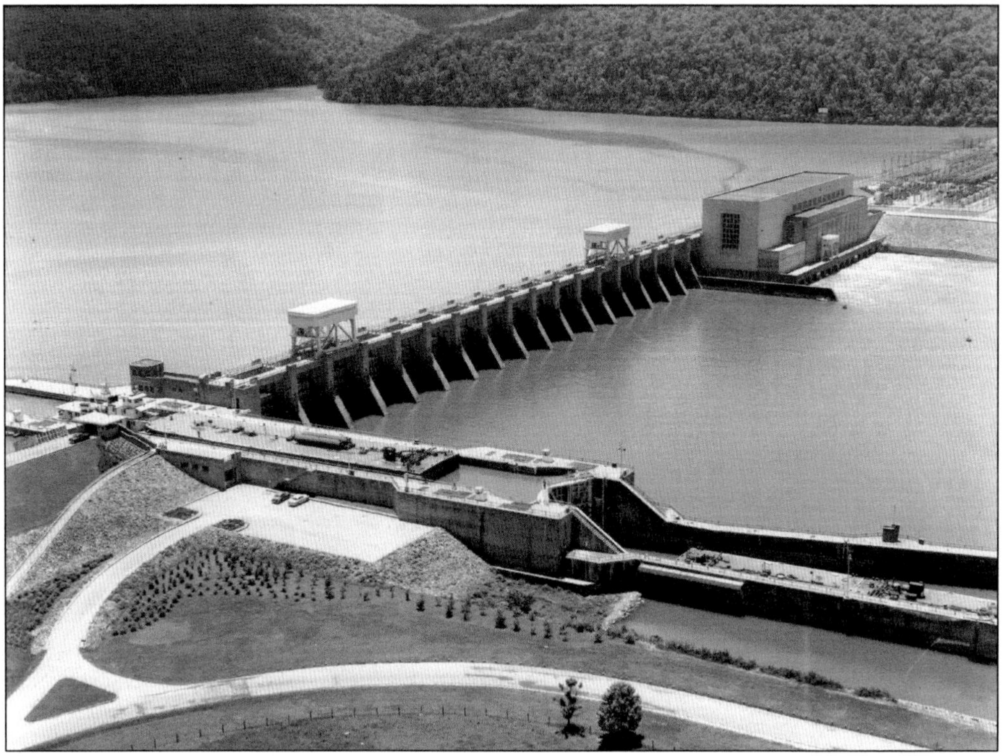

This is the Tennessee Valley Authority Guntersville Dam. Camping, which used to be extremely common to the extent that mere inches separated tents, is no longer allowed. At one point, there was talk of constructing a road across the dam, but US congressman Joe Starnes (D-AL), fearing it might divert traffic from Guntersville, helped squelch the plan. (Guntersville Historical Society.)

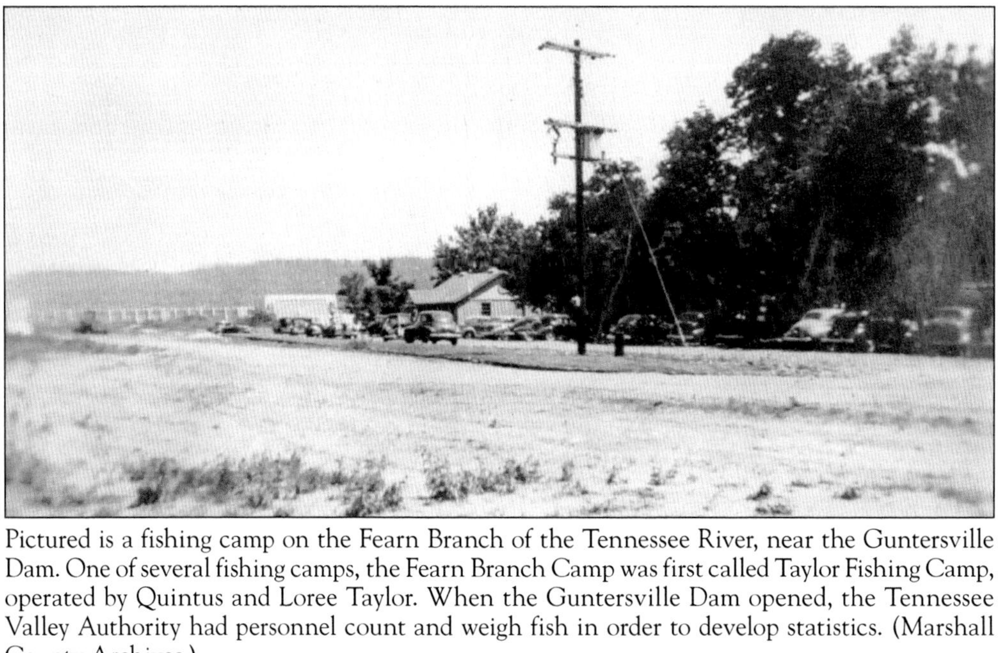

Pictured is a fishing camp on the Fearn Branch of the Tennessee River, near the Guntersville Dam. One of several fishing camps, the Fearn Branch Camp was first called Taylor Fishing Camp, operated by Quintus and Loree Taylor. When the Guntersville Dam opened, the Tennessee Valley Authority had personnel count and weigh fish in order to develop statistics. (Marshall County Archives.)

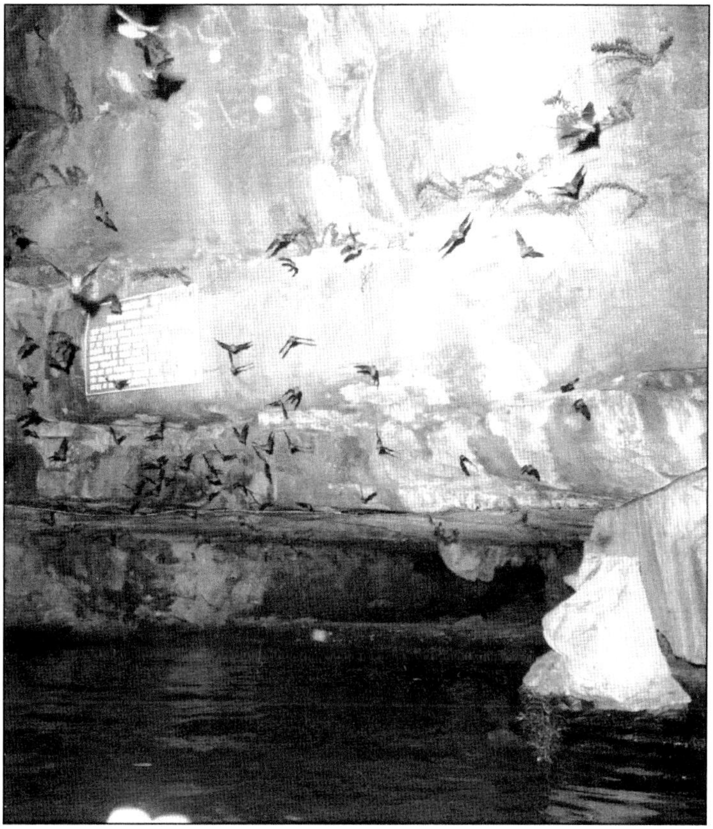

Gray bats are plentiful on Lake Guntersville and frequent its caves, especially Hambrick Cave (locally known as "Bat Cave") above the Tennessee Valley Authority Guntersville Dam. At dusk during summers, kayakers and boaters can witness some 60,000 bats exiting the cave. No visitors are allowed in the cave, a point made clear by signs and a fence. (*Advertiser-Gleam*.)

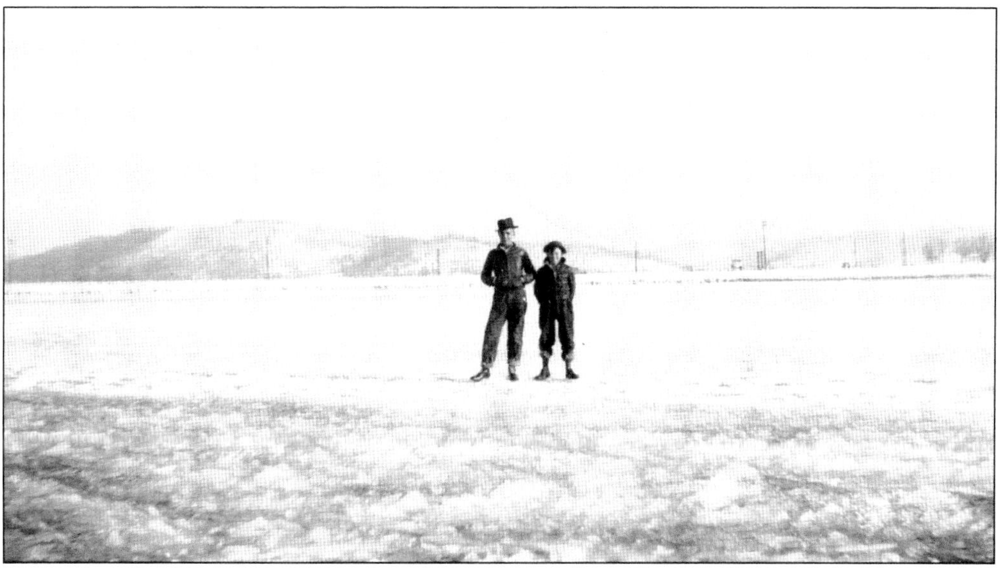

These two unidentified boys are standing on Lake Guntersville when it partially froze in 1940. The temperature had hovered around 0 degrees Fahrenheit for some days, and the winter had been harsh, with some 10 inches of snow. Roger Hyde, Ralph Cornelius, and Bill Harris braved the ice and walked about a mile. Martha Bradford was the only woman known to have ventured onto the ice. (Nancy Gilbreath Graham.)

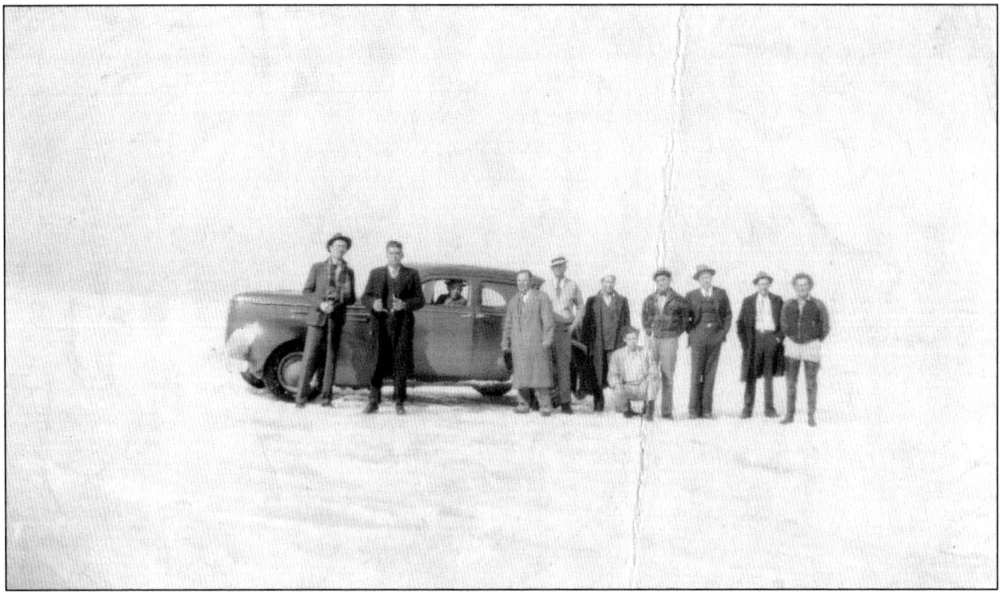

This 1940 photograph is of a 4,600-pound 1939 Studebaker President driven 200 feet onto the frozen lake by Howard Powell Sr. (in car). Also pictured are, from left to right, J.L. Hartley, Buster Alred, Jess Duncan, Rader Sayer, Cecil Cotton, Buddy Powell, John Oaks, Red Barksdale, Oliver Campbell, and Marvin Denham. (Nancy Gilbreath Graham.)

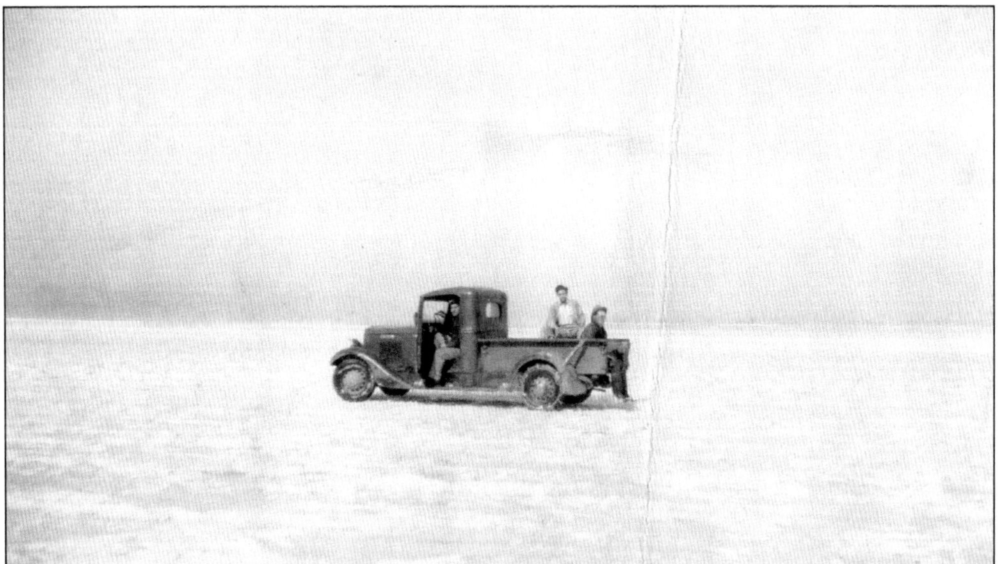

This truck was driven 250 feet onto the frozen Lake Guntersville in 1940. From left to right are John Oaks, Buddy Powell, and Marvin Denham. Oaks had borrowed the truck from his employer, the Bush Motor Company. The lake was frozen some six inches in places. Steamboats were impeded, and a Nashville, Chattanooga & St. Louis Railway boat used its stern to break the ice. (Nancy Gilbreath Graham.)

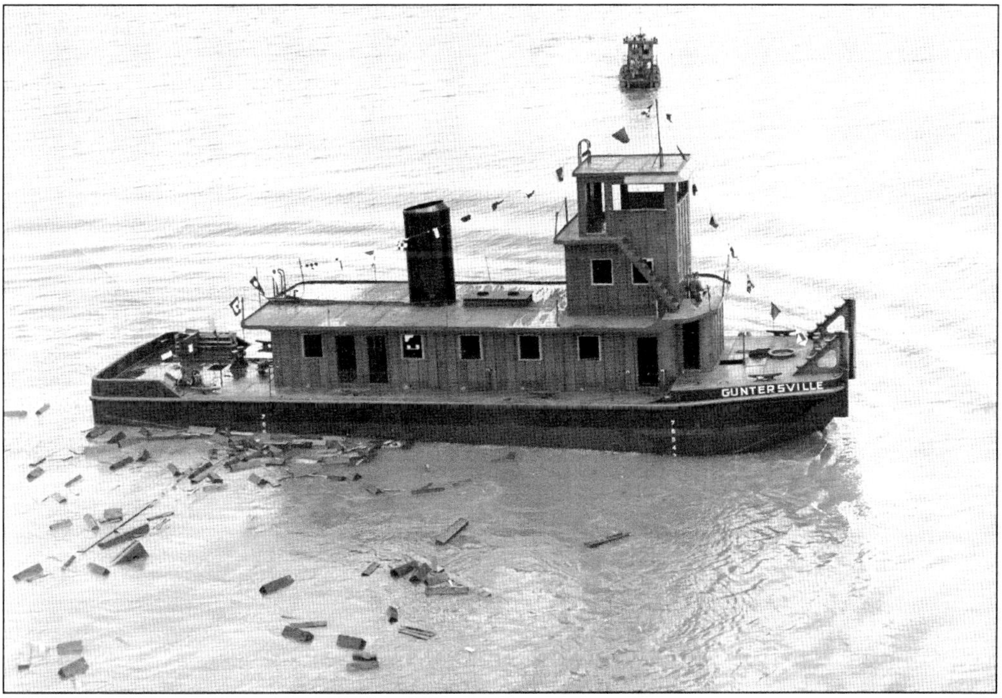

On June 13, 1946, *Miss Guntersville* (pictured) was launched. With the creation of the lake, Guntersville began seeing extensive barge traffic. In 1943, G.N. Robertson, owner of the Robertson Line, sent the tugboat *Afres* from Indiana to be stationed in Guntersville. Over the years, several other tugboats, like *Gary* and *Huntsville*, operated in Guntersville. (Guntersville Museum.)

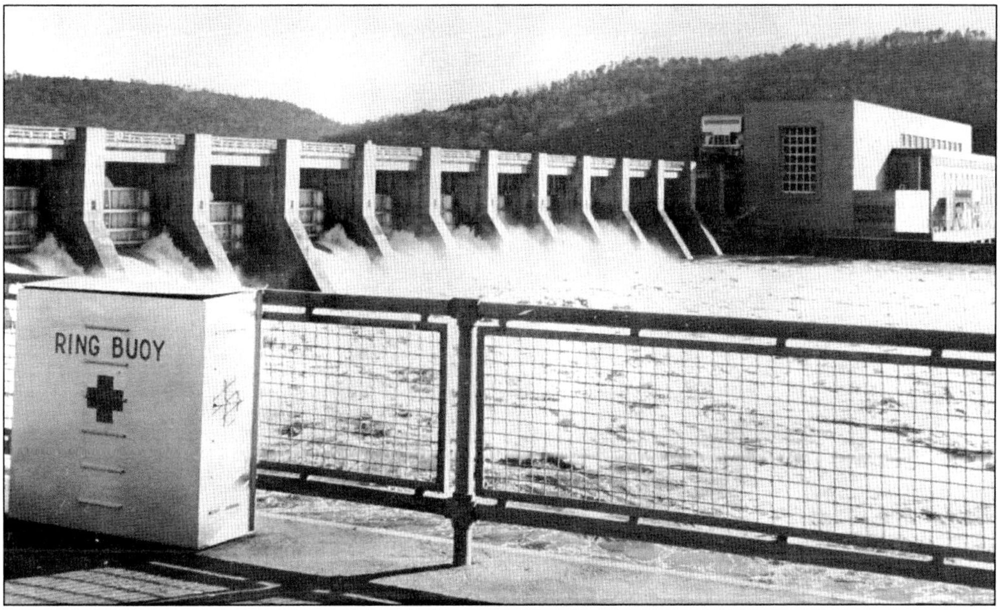

This c. 1950s picture of Guntersville Dam shows the floodgates. Below the dam is a sandbar that is popular with fishermen and lure seekers. Indeed, a veritable treasure trove of lead and various types of fishing tackle can be found buried in the sand or wedged under rocks and boulders when the floodgates close. (Mike Jones.)

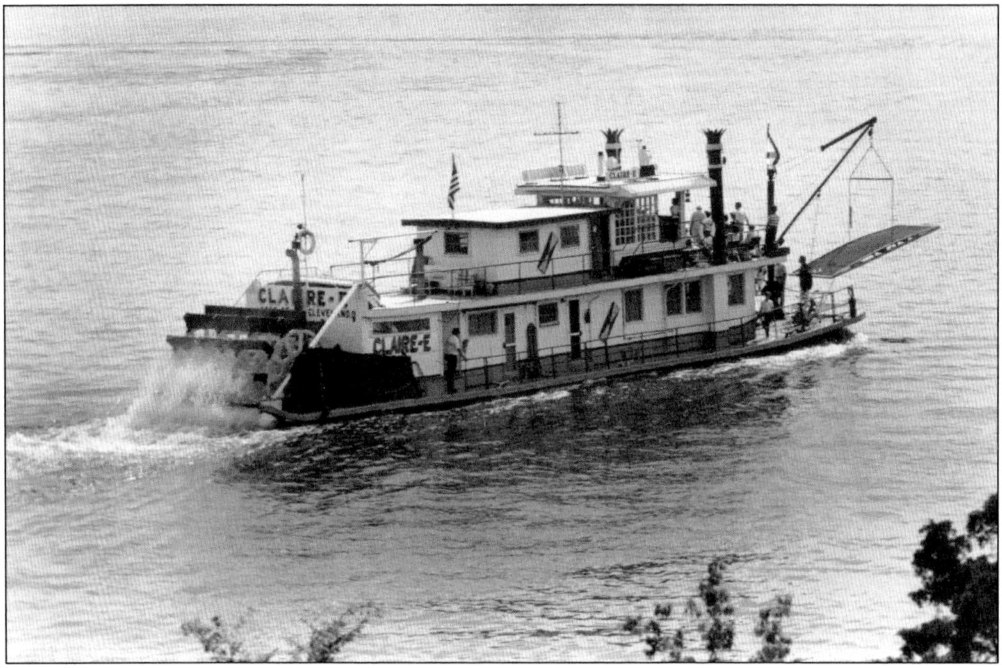

This is the *Claire-E* stern-wheeler on Lake Guntersville. It was built in 1926 and was in a variety of cities. It spent 13 years in Guntersville. Gene and Claire Fitch purchased the boat and made their home on it in the late 1960s. The boat weighed 100 tons and was 115 feet by 18 feet. (*Advertiser-Gleam*.)

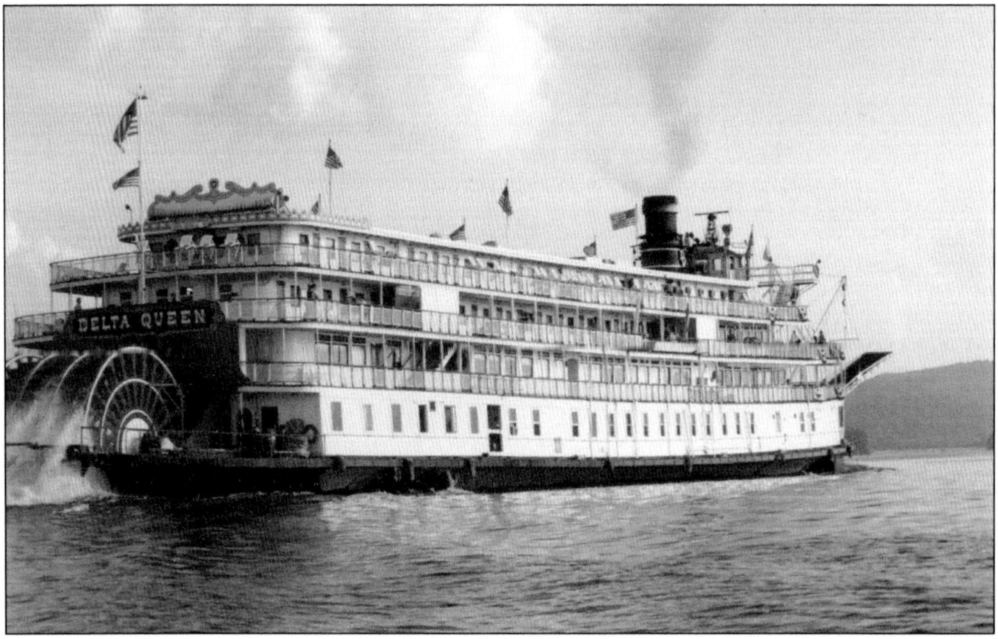

The *Delta Queen* steamboat, built in 1926, is shown. It visited Guntersville a few times over the decades. It gained popularity by providing tourist cruises all along the Mississippi and Tennessee Rivers as well as tributaries. The famous steamboat is a National Historic Landmark and also listed in the National Register of Historic Places. (Buddy Taylor.)

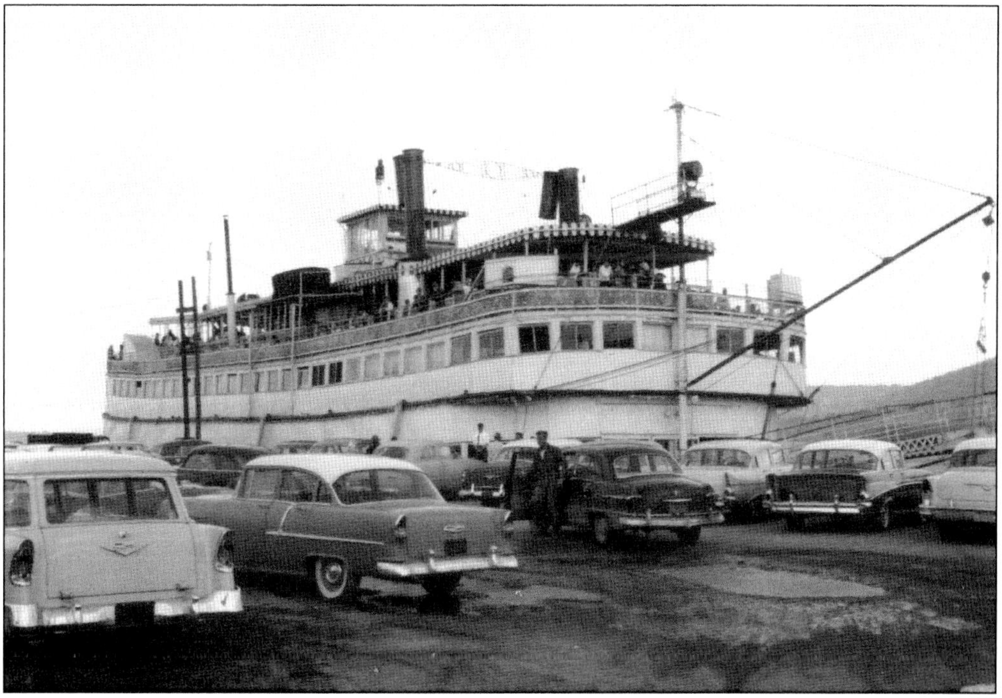

This is the *Avalon*, a steamboat docked at the Guntersville Harbor, around the early 1950s. It began as a ferry but in 1930 was made into a cruiser. In 1952 alone, it traveled roughly 9,000 miles throughout the Ohio, Mississippi, and Tennessee Rivers. It had four decks, a steel hull, and was 181 by 57 feet. (Gail Smith Ingrum.)

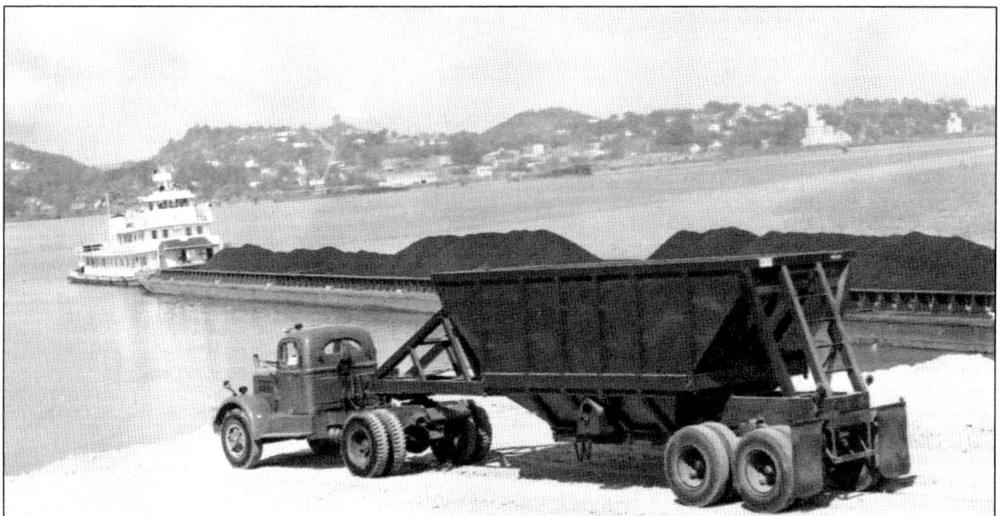

In 1953, Guntersville's port had barges arrive with coal, which was then hauled on specially designed trucks to Rome, Georgia, for Georgia Power's steam plant. Each truck made four round-trips a day, with 18 tons per trip. The trucks operated 20 hours a day with two shifts. The Coal Transfer Company was a subsidiary of Chatham Transportation Company of Atlanta. (Larry Smith.)

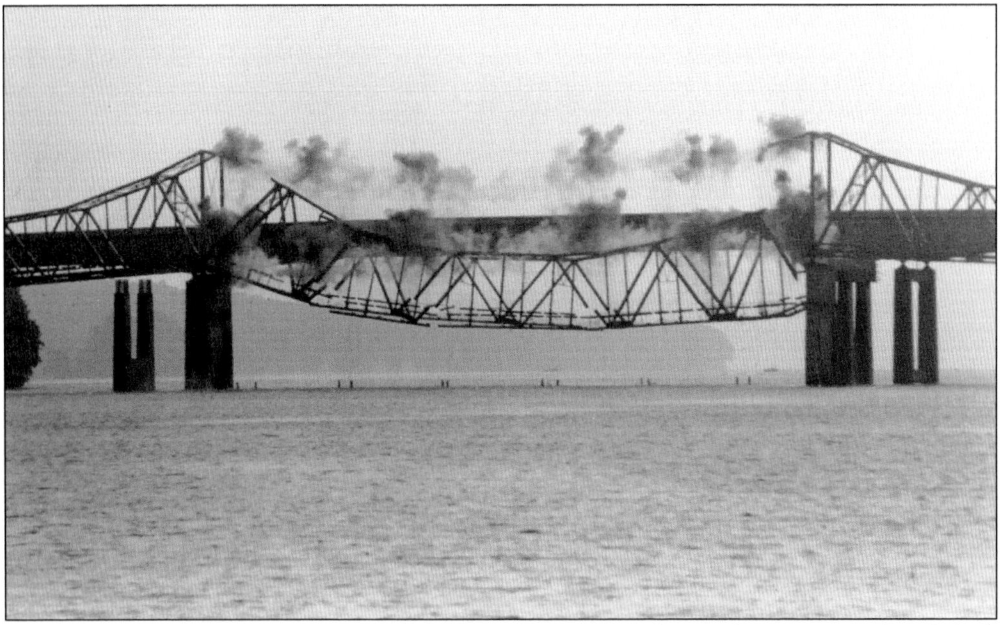

In 1992, the George Houston Bridge, originally built in 1928 and opened in 1930, was demolished, much to the dismay of Kermit Scheer, who headed a Save the Bridge campaign. He and roughly 2,000 supporters had hoped the bridge might be left standing as a place to walk and fish. In his words, "Think of what a tourist attraction that old bridge could have been." (*Advertiser-Gleam.*)

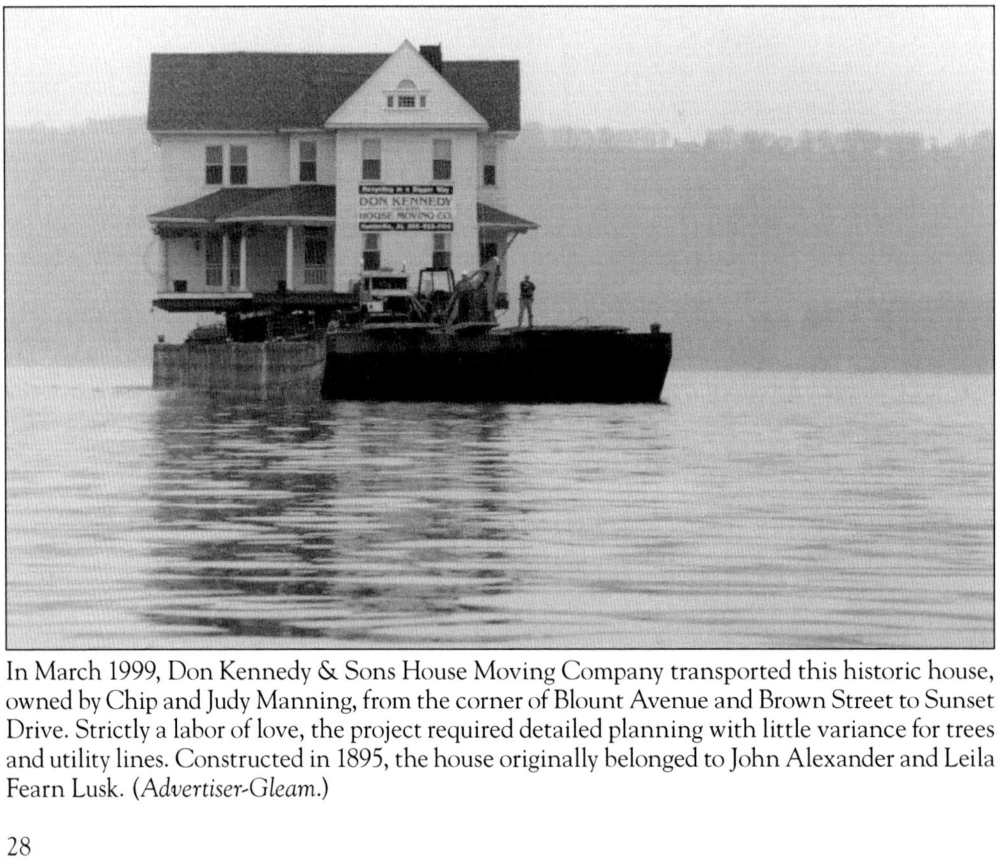

In March 1999, Don Kennedy & Sons House Moving Company transported this historic house, owned by Chip and Judy Manning, from the corner of Blount Avenue and Brown Street to Sunset Drive. Strictly a labor of love, the project required detailed planning with little variance for trees and utility lines. Constructed in 1895, the house originally belonged to John Alexander and Leila Fearn Lusk. (*Advertiser-Gleam.*)

Two

Beauty Pageants

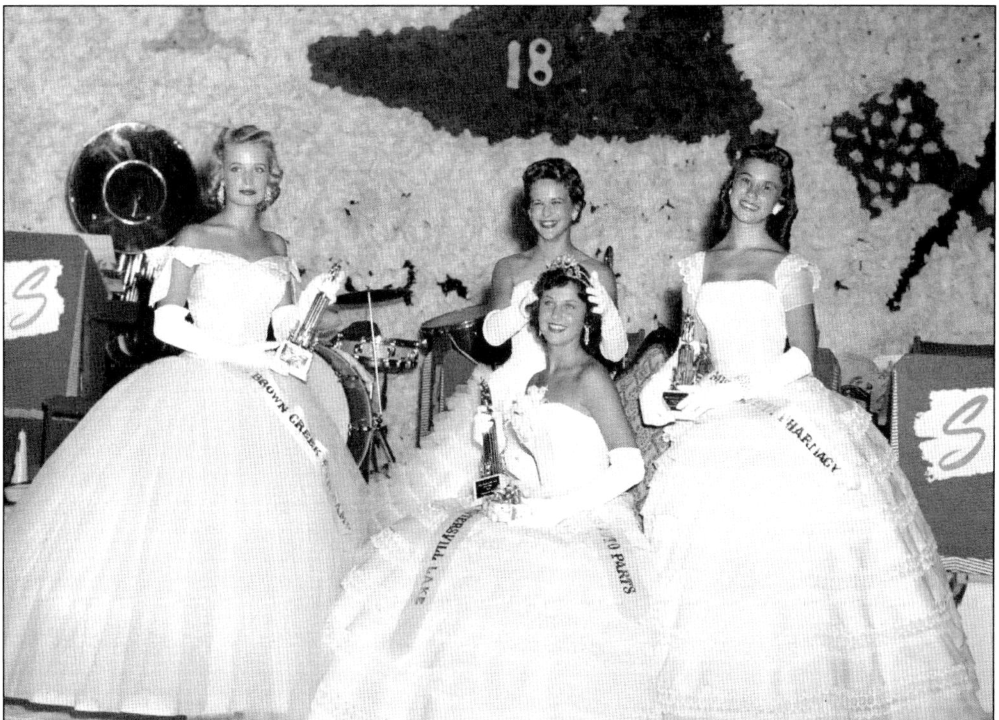

Seated is Boaz's Frances Wells (Miss Guntersville Lake 1957) and standing, from left to right, are Betty Lindstrom (second place), Sarah Jane Mabrey (Miss Guntersville Lake 1956), and Dorothy Jo Oaks (third place). While this pageant lasted until the late 1980s, only six of the first-place winners were natives of Guntersville. (Marshall County Archives.)

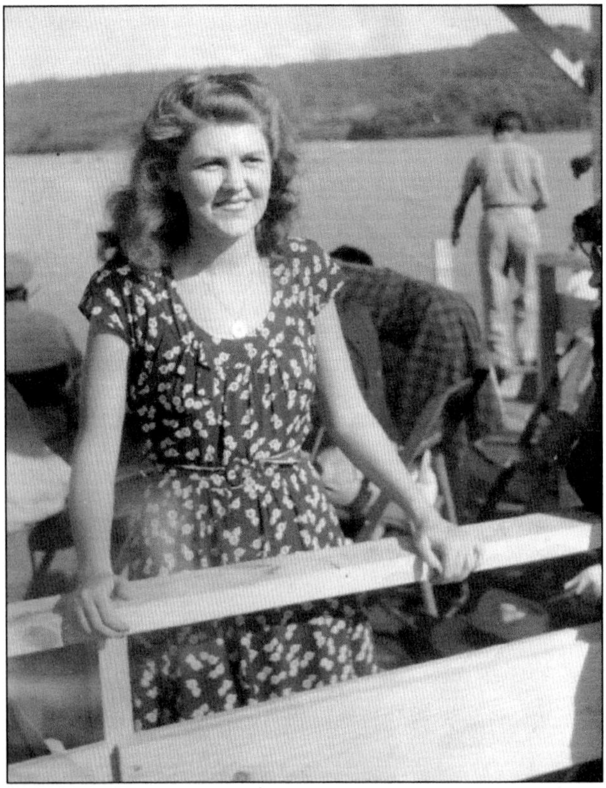

This is Ida Will Willis, the first Miss Guntersville Lake. Even though the boat races began in 1939, the beauty pageant did not become a part of the festivities until 1946. Local businesses sponsored 51 girls in the 1946 contest. The boat races that year earned a $3,000 profit, which the community used on the next year's race. (Gail Smith Ingrum.)

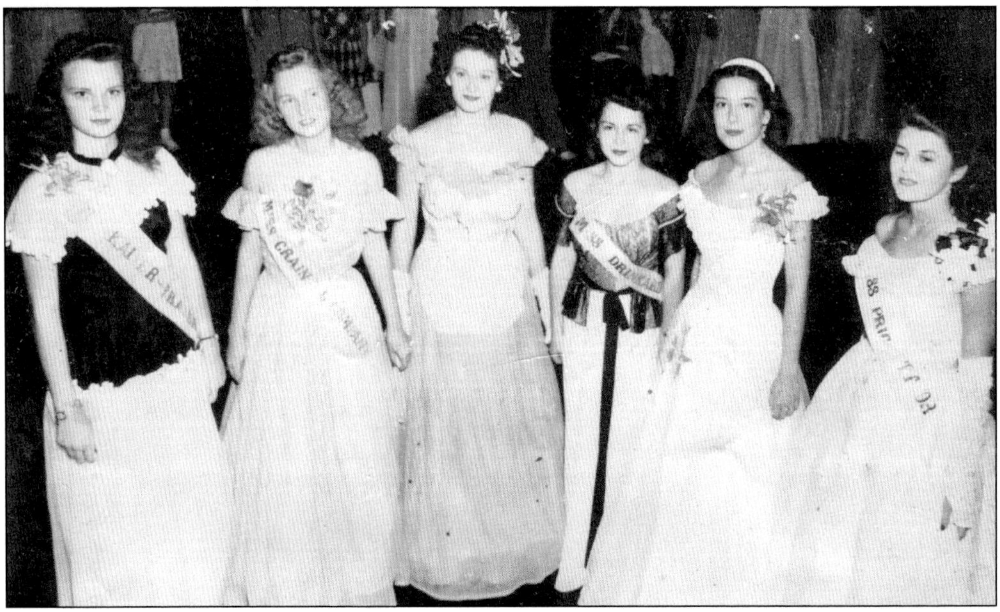

From left to right are unidentified, Jan Albert, Margaret Brown, Frances Slayton, Joy Conard, and Ida Will Willis. Gov. James "Big Jim" Folsom crowned Willis and even kissed her. Ida Will Willis married Claude Herbert Smith; they lived in Guntersville for many years but later moved to Tennessee. They maintained a home, the White Elephant, in Guntersville. (Marshall County Archives.)

Alabama governor James "Big Jim" Folsom is shown dancing with Ida Will Willis. Willis's father kept a close eye on the governor, who was also nicknamed "Kissin' Jim." Folsom, who had a home in nearby Cullman, often attended the boat races, because he was quite fond of Guntersville and kept a cabin on the lake for his family. (Gail Smith Ingrum.)

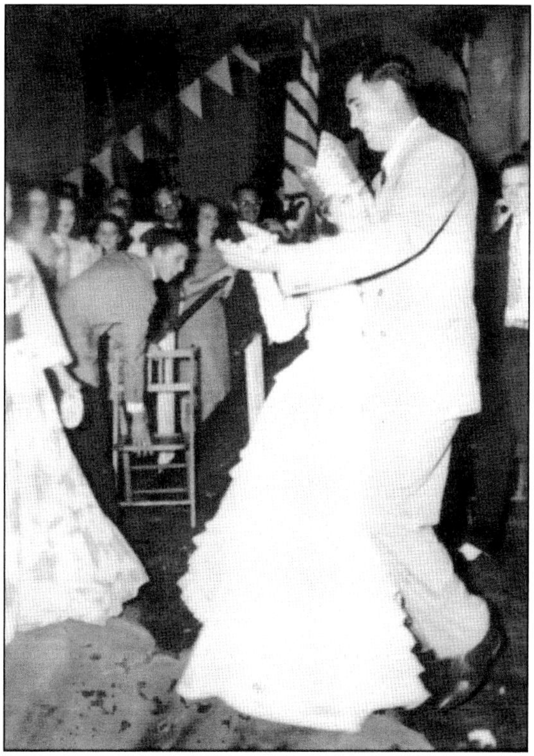

This is a photograph of the Guntersville Shriners around the late 1940s with nine beauty contestants in the background. The women are, from left to right, (first row) Peggy McLemore, Maureen Gore, Martha Nell Rains, Jan Albert, and Helen Gilbreath, (second row) Dot Kilcrease, Martha Walker, Lamb Rayburn, and Margaret Brown Henderson. (Gail Smith Ingrum.)

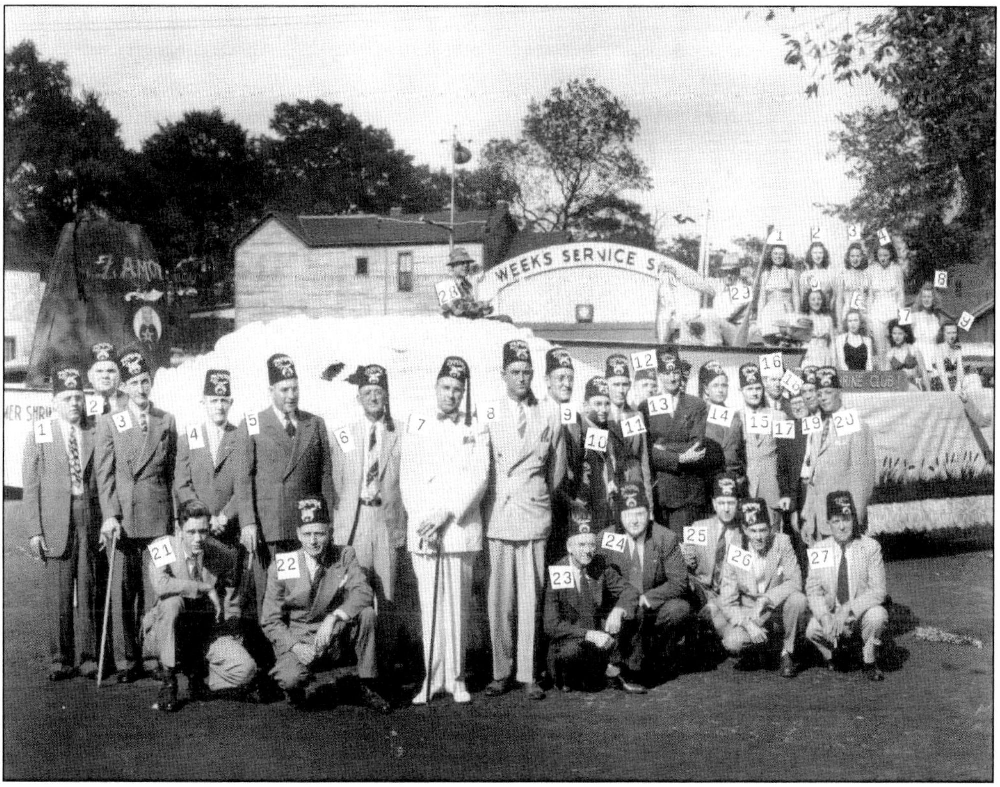

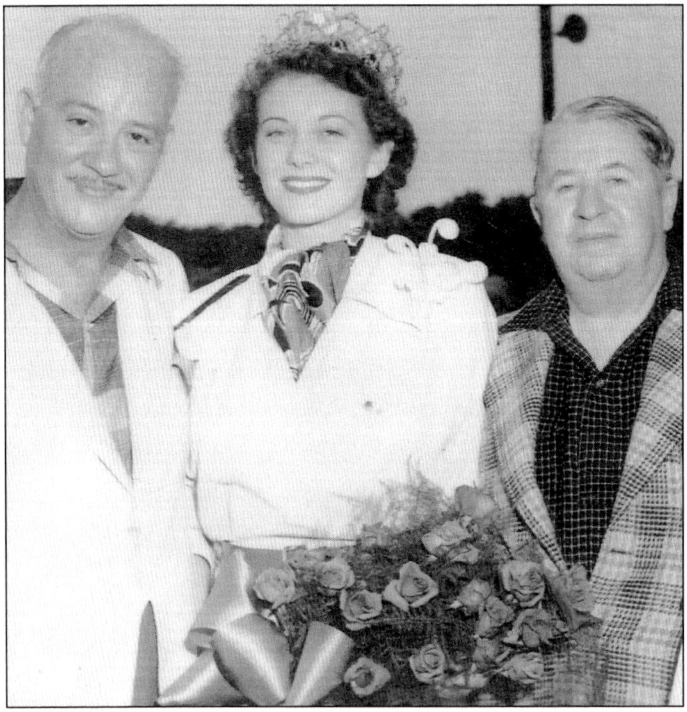

Guntersville native Margaret Brown (center), Miss Guntersville Lake 1948, is posing with two reporters from the *Tennessean*. Since its inception in 1946, the pageant had been limited to contestants from Marshall County. In 1948, the contest was opened to all Alabama women as long as they were 15–25 years old, single, and sponsored by a Guntersville business. (Guntersville Museum.)

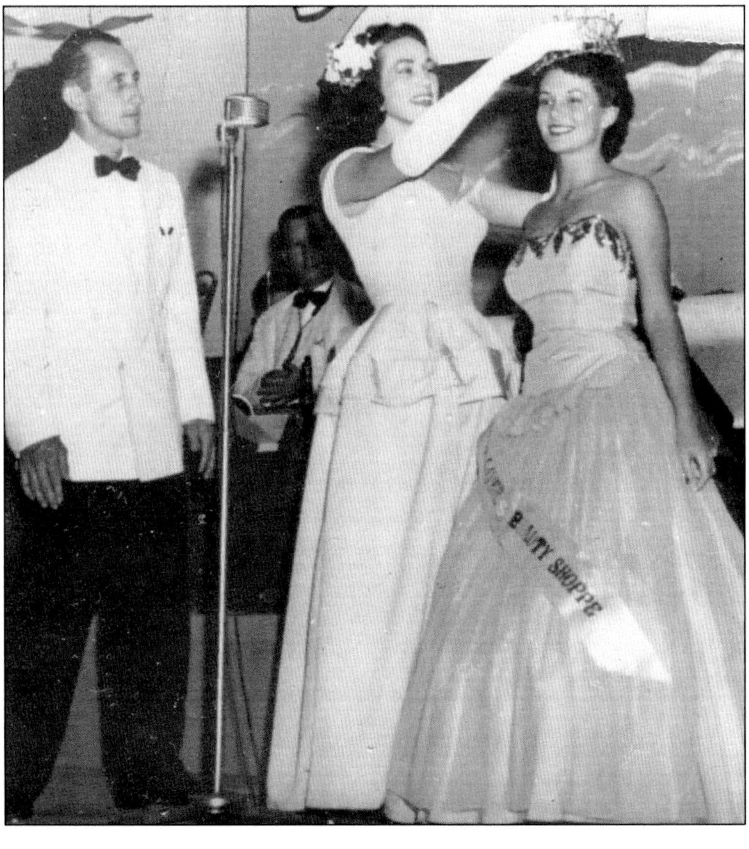

Pictured, from left to right, are emcee Bookie Coplin, Martha Ann Ingram (Miss Guntersville Lake 1947), and Margaret Brown (Miss Guntersville Lake 1948). Mary Elizabeth Long won second place, and Martha Kelley won third place. Ingram, from Tarrant City, won Miss Alabama in 1948 and also competed in the Miss America contest. (Marshall County Archives.)

On August 7, 1948, the second Little Miss Guntersville Lake pageant took place with 40 girls vying for the title. From left to right are Linda Ann Scruggs of Fort Payne (winner), Kay Martin (second place), and Nancy Jane Coplin (third place). One of the judges was Harry Brundidge, a writer for *Cosmopolitan*. (Marshall County Archives.)

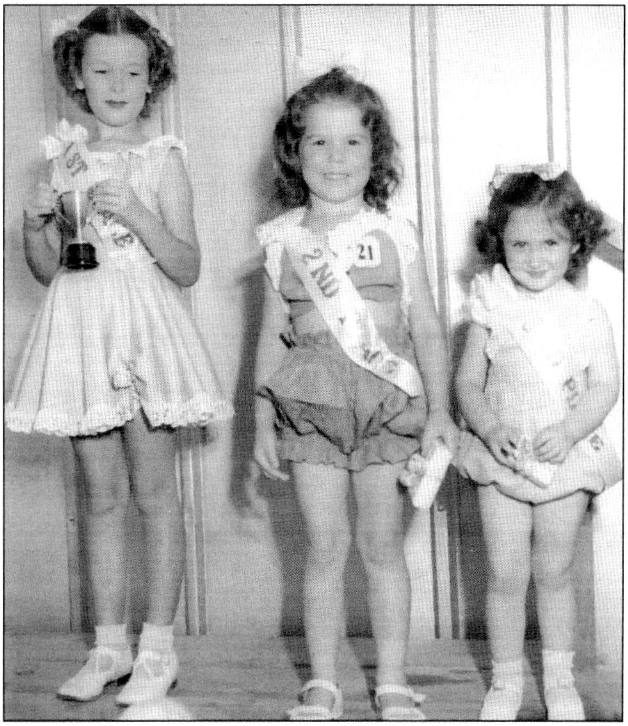

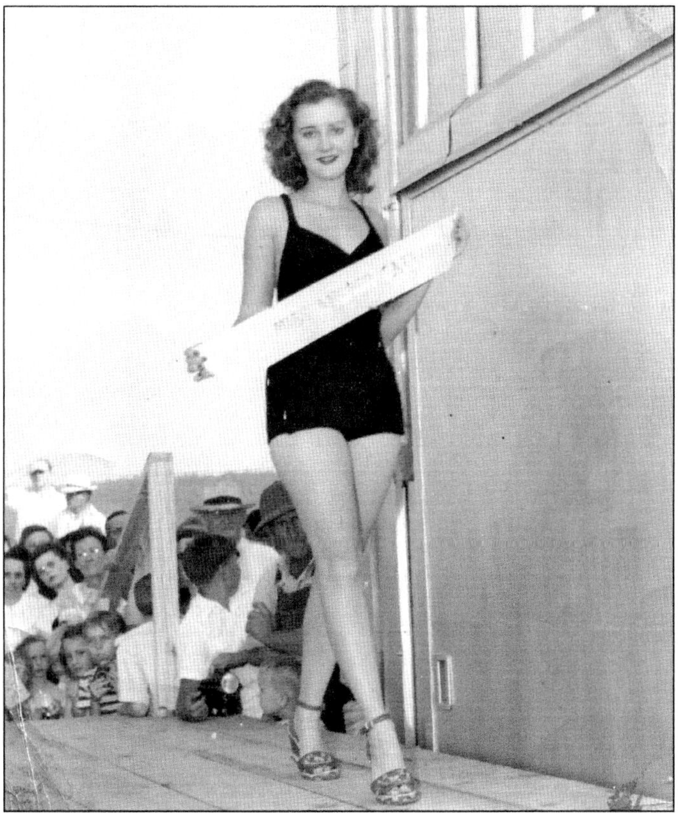

This is Bobbie Conner, a contestant in the 1948 and 1949 Miss Guntersville Lake pageant. "I do not even recall who won either year but it was more about fun and participating in all the party environment or hoopla that it entailed for Guntersville." The bathing suit category took place at the yacht club, while the evening wear category transpired at the armory. (Bobbie Conner Curry.)

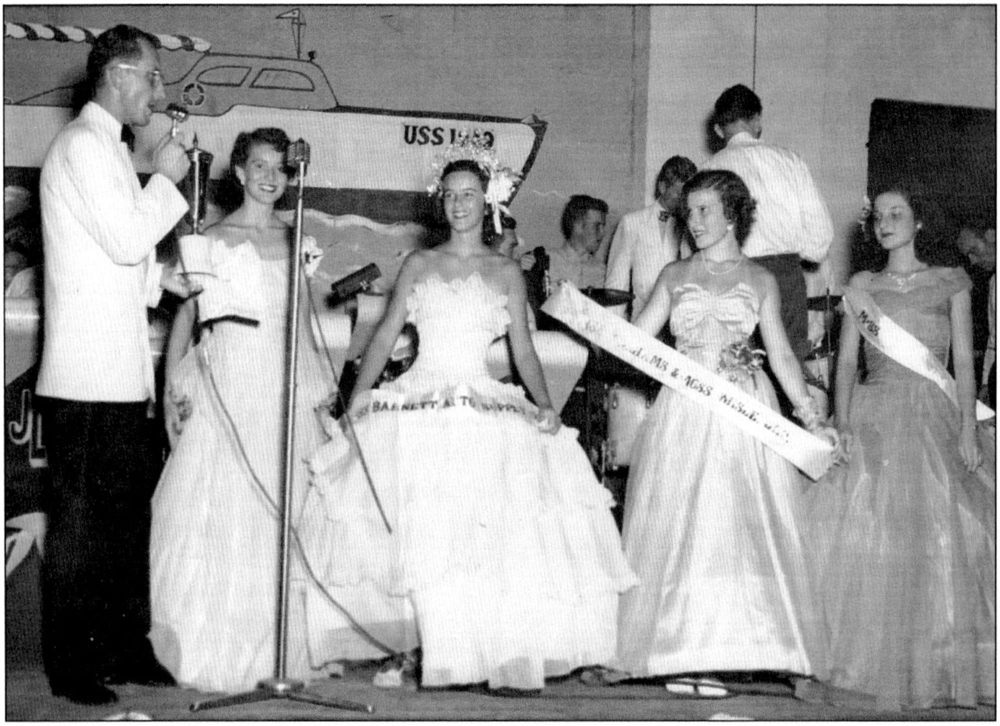

Above, from left to right, are Bookie Coplin (emcee), Margaret Brown (Miss Guntersville Lake 1948), Patsy Hill (Miss Guntersville Lake 1949), Johnny Long (orchestra leader), Claudette Long (second place), and Fran King (third place). According to pageant chair Elsie Crain, "The beauty contest plays a vital part in helping to put over the [boat] races and advertise Guntersville." (Marshall County Archives.)

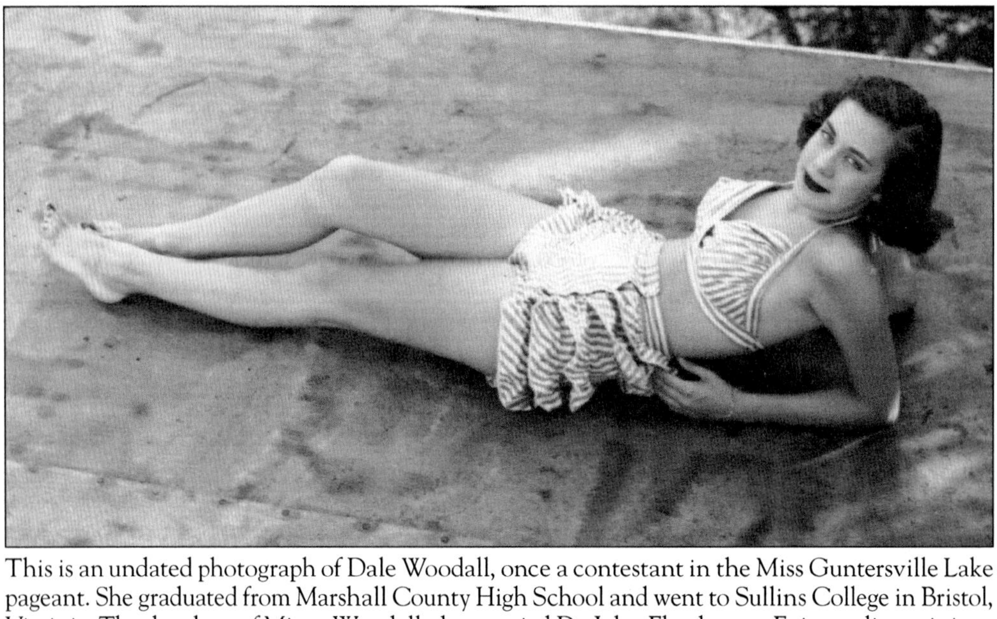

This is an undated photograph of Dale Woodall, once a contestant in the Miss Guntersville Lake pageant. She graduated from Marshall County High School and went to Sullins College in Bristol, Virginia. The daughter of Minor Woodall, she married Dr. John Fletcher, an Episcopalian minister and brother of Academy Award–winning actress Louise Fletcher. (Marshall County Archives.)

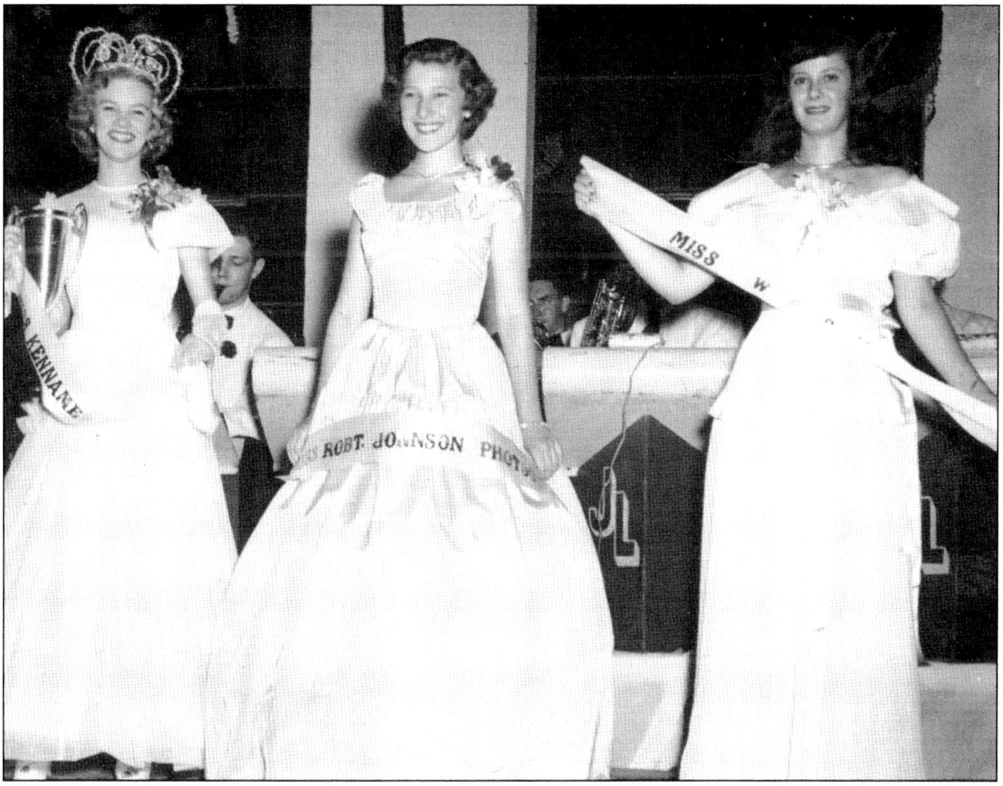

From left to right are Mary Elizabeth Patterson (Miss Guntersville Lake 1950), Claudette Long (second place), and Betty Sue Woods (third place). Patterson reflected that during the bathing suit portion of the contest, she winked at a friend and, to her shock, suddenly realized that one of the judges thought the gesture directed at him. In her words, "I couldn't help but laugh." (Marshall County Archives.)

Contestants in the Little Miss Guntersville Lake pageant had to live in or near Guntersville or their parents had to have a cabin or boat on the lake. Thirty girls competed in the 1950 contest, and the winners, shown from left to right, were Mary Lane Moss (third place), Judy Page Clayton (second place), and Sharon Drinkard (first place). (Marshall County Archives.)

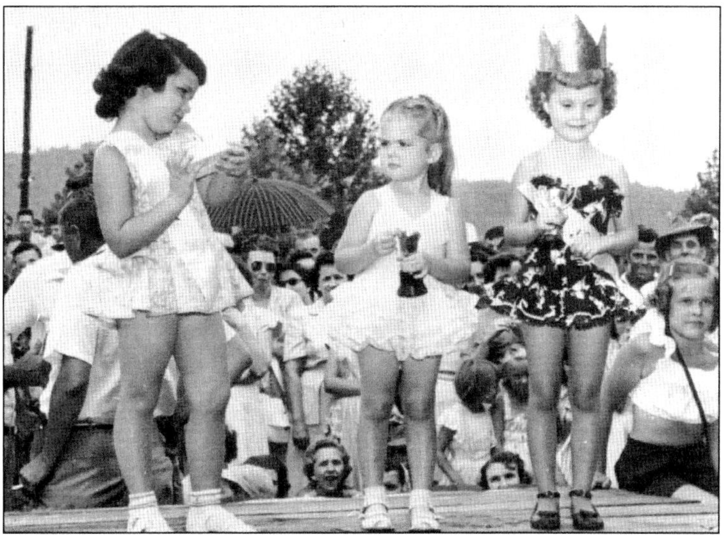

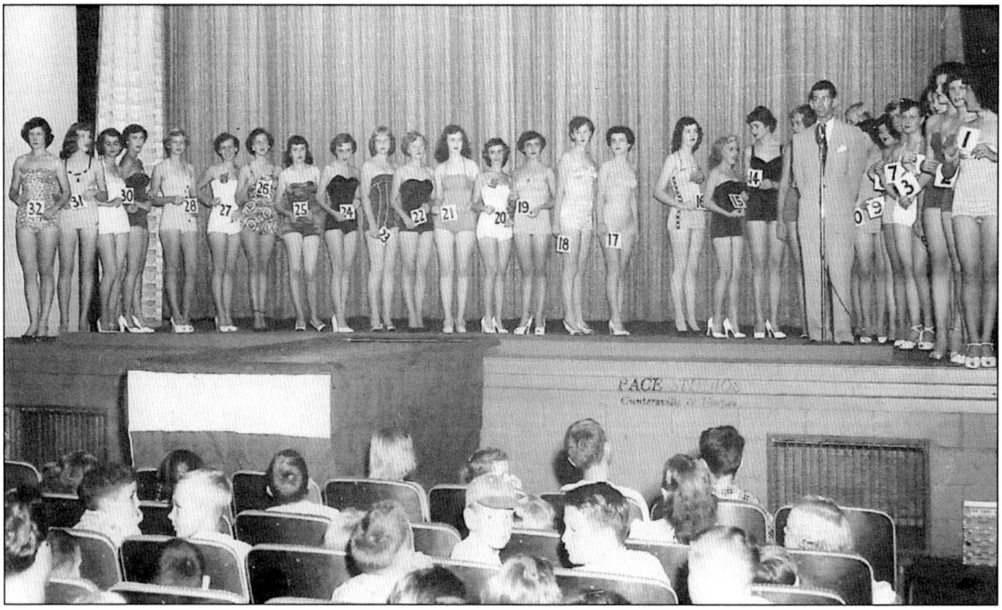

These are some of the contestants in the 1952 Miss Marshall County pageant: Ann Todd (8), Doris Jean Kellar (13), Mary Ruth McClendon (14), Bonnie Smith (15), Lena Kate Hodges (19), Barbara Ann Sims (20), Marguerite Moon (23), Betty Jean Boyce (30), Mary Carmen Burt (31), and Barbara Ann Jackson (32). The winner was Sims. Ray McClendon is at the microphone. (Guntersville Historical Society.)

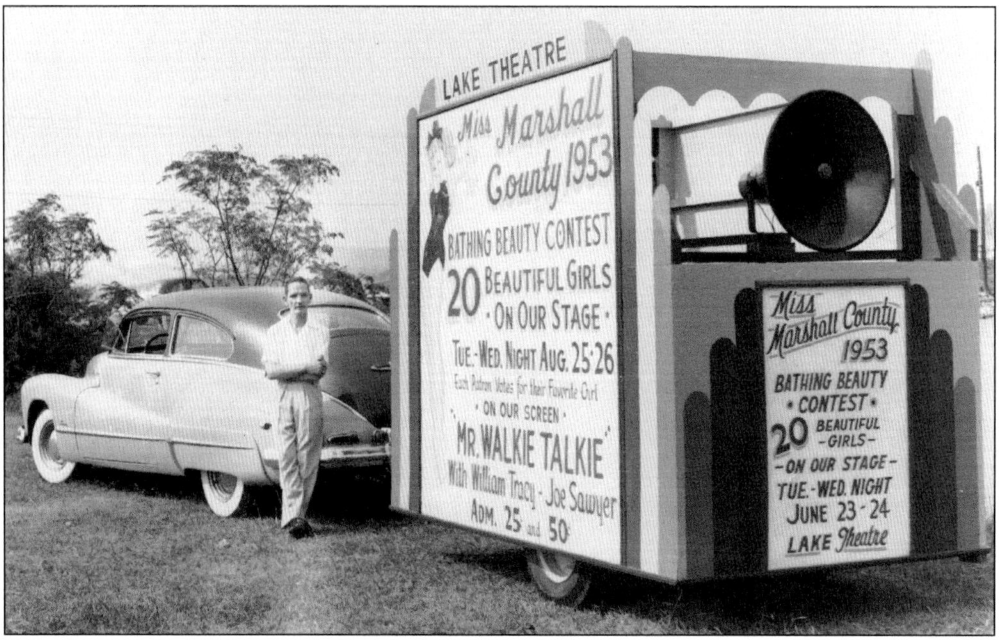

Bill Harris (pictured), manager of the Lake Theatre, heavily advertised the 1953 Miss Marshall County pageant. The sign on the side of the trailer reads, "Bathing beauty contest; 20 beautiful girls on our stage; Tue-Wed night Aug 25-26; each patron votes for their favorite girl; on our screen: 'Mr. Walkie Talkie' with William Tracy [and] Joe Sawyer; Admission 25¢ and 50¢." (Nancy Gilbreath Graham.)

Nancy Lay became Miss Marshall County in 1953. Of the other contestants that year, the following were from Guntersville: Louise Elliott (second), Betty Boyce, Nira Smith, Betty Ann Whitworth, Margaret Walker, and Dell Whitehead. The pageant was held at the Lake Theatre and, as always, attracted an audience. (Marshall County Archives.)

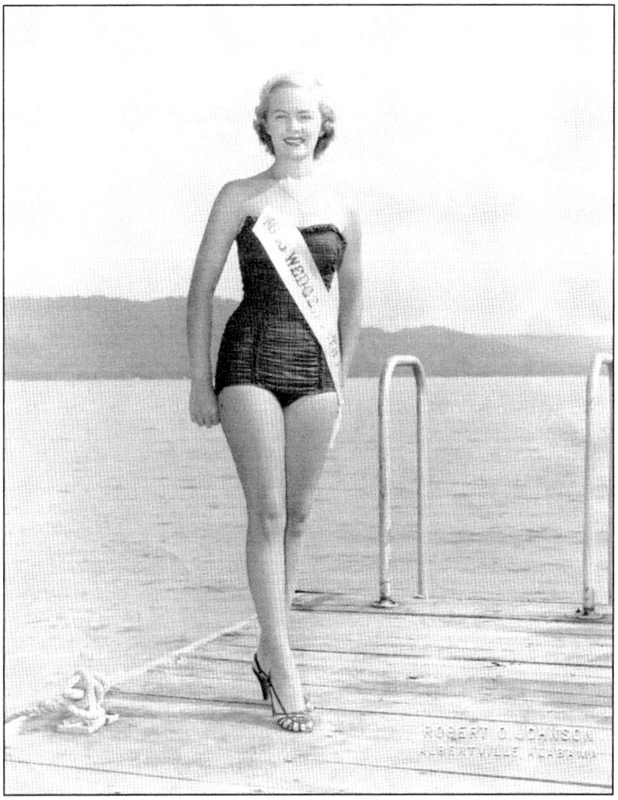

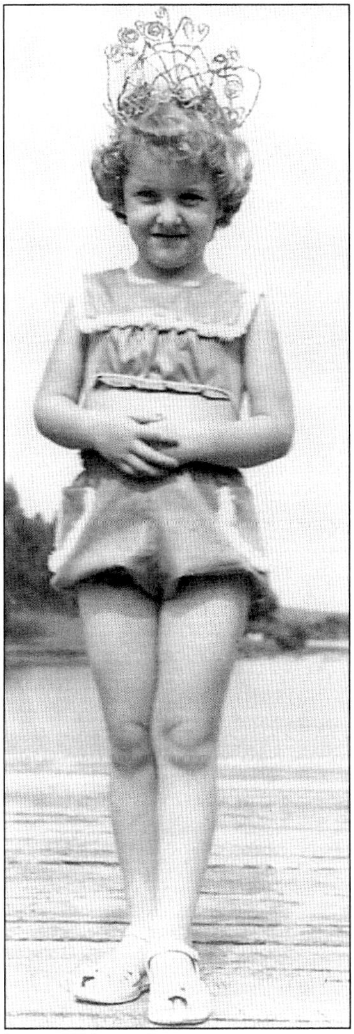

This is Gail Smith, who became Little Miss Guntersville Lake in 1953. She is the daughter of Claude Herbert Smith and Ida Will Willis. Cynthia Hubble won second place, and Beverly Lynn won third place. Judges were Bill Johnson (New Orleans, Louisiana), Ed Endres (Buffalo, New York), and Steve Flowers (Port Arthur, Texas). (Gail Smith Ingrum.)

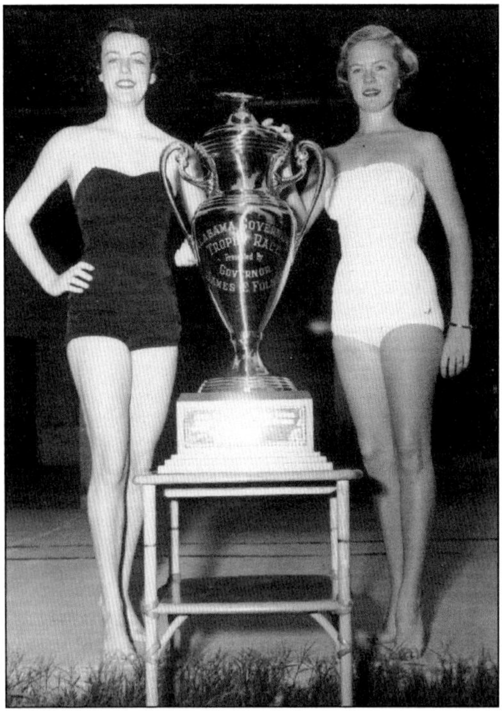

Guntersville girls Jane Haralson (left) and Nancy Lay are posing with the 1955 Alabama Governor's Trophy, which was donated by Gov. James "Big Jim" Folsom. Several other pageant contestants, including Karen Kirk, Margie Kirk, and Prissy Dunson, had their pictures taken with the trophy that year. The trophy is currently in the possession of the Guntersville Museum. (Marshall County Archives.)

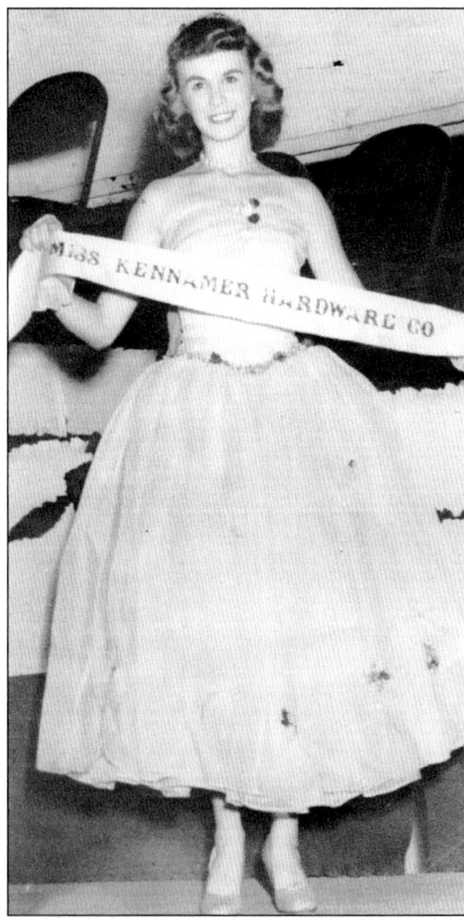

Shown is Barbara Ann Sims, a contestant in the 1955 Miss Guntersville Lake pageant. That year, while appearing on Arthur Godfrey's television show, bandleader Guy Lombardo mentioned being a fan of the Guntersville boat races. While primarily known for his musical skills, Lombardo was a devoted hydroplane racer and boating enthusiast. (Gail Smith Ingrum.)

This is Guntersville native Mary "Tootsie" Rains, a contestant in the 1955 Miss Guntersville Lake pageant. Arab entries were Mary Jo Camp and Ruth Copeland. Albertville entries were Wanda Smith, Judy Holder, and Joyce Jenkins. Boaz entries were Judy Thrasher, Elizabeth Thrasher, and Sarah Bruce. (Marshall County Archives.)

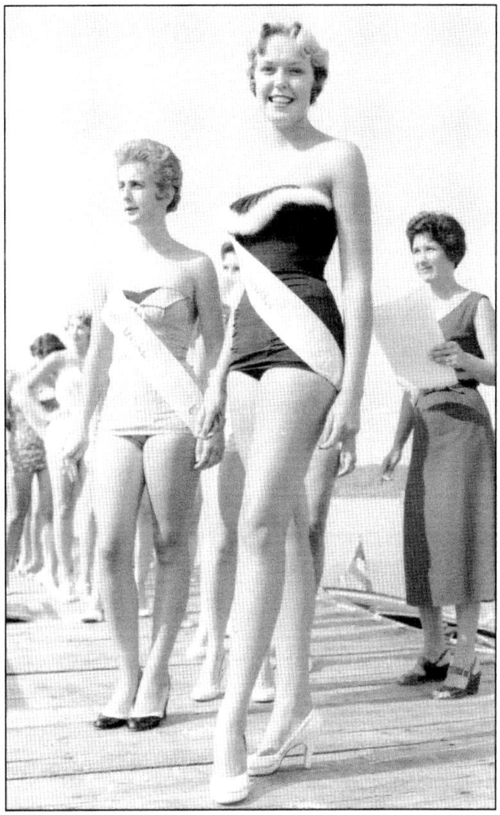

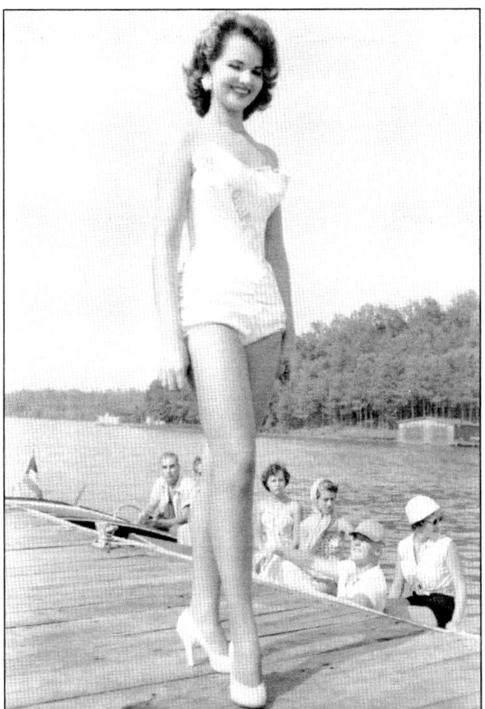

Shown is Patsy Elliott (Miss Guntersville Lake 1955) of Tarrant City. Among the Guntersville girls competing that year were Carolyn Cornelius, Nancy Grant, Celia Norris Martin, Gail Whitmire, Barbara Ann Sims, Kay McCormick, Jane Haralson, Margie Kirk, Ann Hunt, Joan Purser, and Karen Kirk. (Marshall County Archives.)

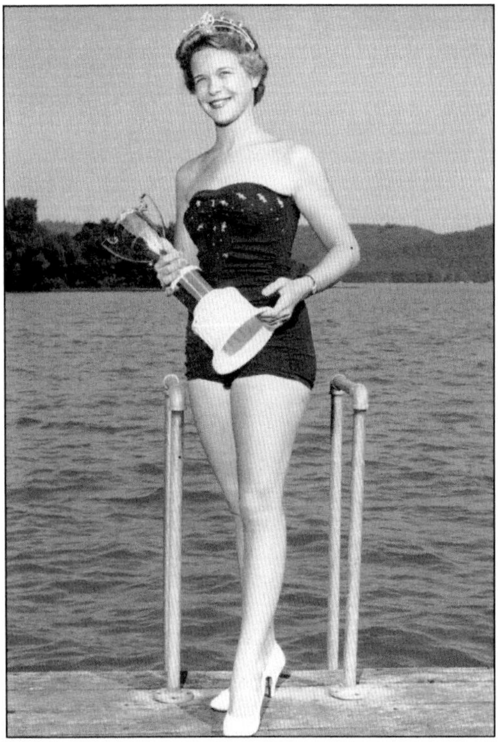

This is Sarah Jane Mabrey (Miss Guntersville Lake 1956). In her words, "I am especially glad to have had a part in the boat race program because the Jaycees have done so much for the teenagers here in the way of better recreation. This was one of the reasons so many of the Guntersville girls were glad to take part in the contest." (Marshall County Archives.)

From left to right are contestants in a Miss Guntersville Lake pageant around 1956: Patricia Patterson, Sally Scott, Sarah Jane Mabrey, Oma Jane Rogers, Jo Ann Moore, Jane Haralson, Karen Drinkard, Charlene Raley, Carolyn Cornelius, Dorothy Jo Oaks, and Dianne Richter. (Marshall County Archives.)

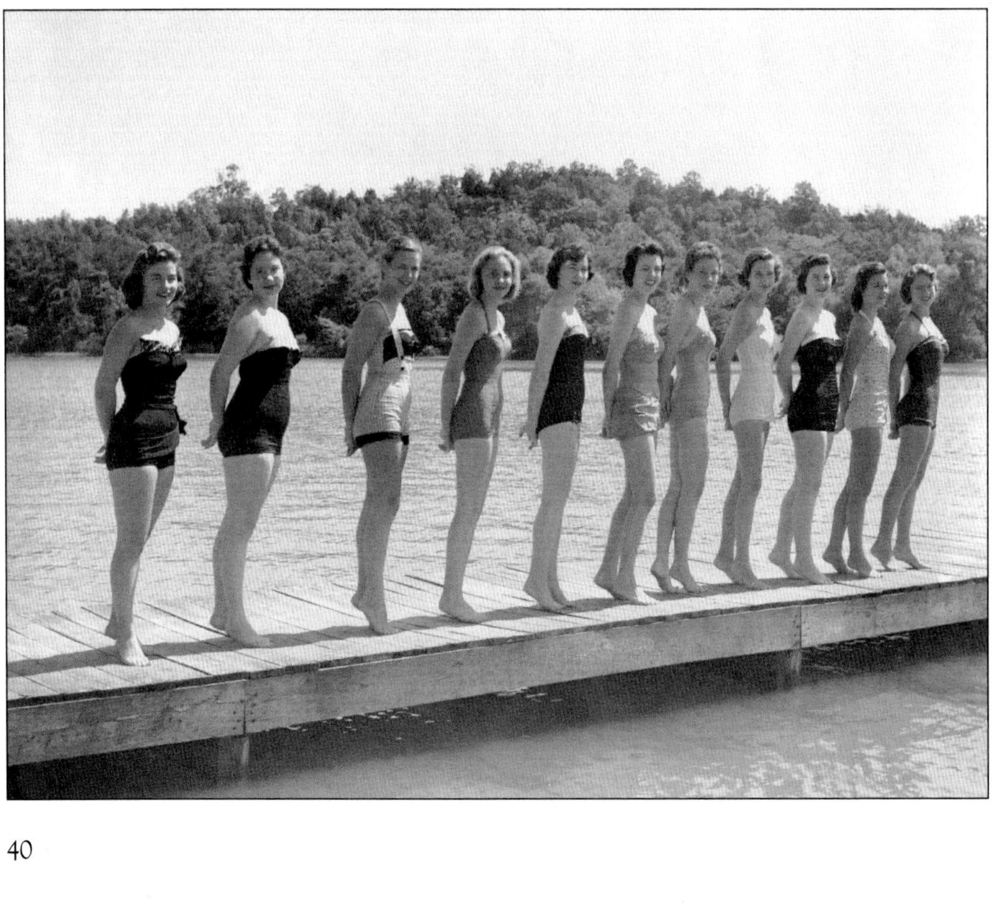

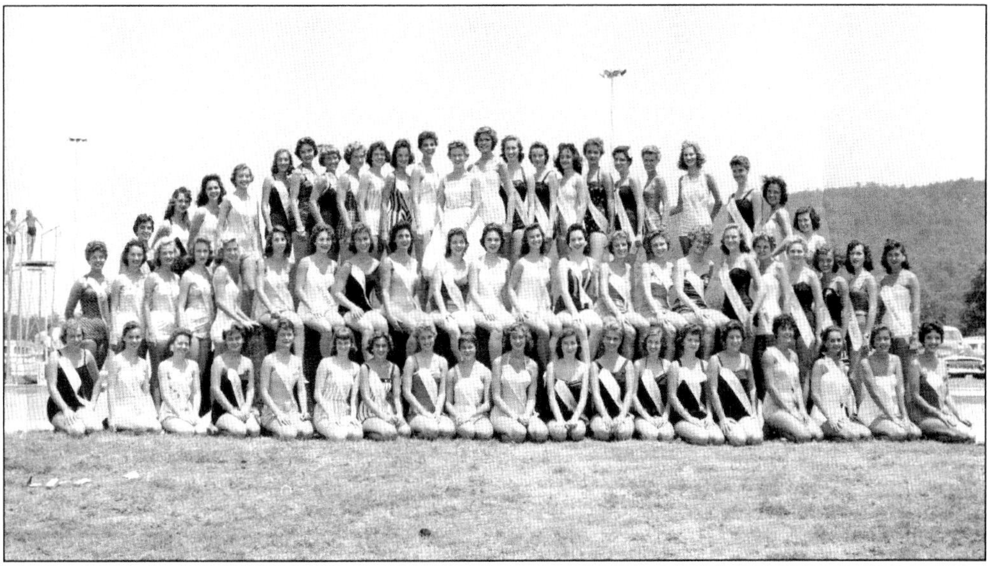

Shown are Miss Guntersville Lake contestants in 1957. Sarah Jane Mabrey (Miss Guntersville Lake 1956) is in the middle of the last row. That year, the bathing suit competition took place at Val Monte Shores resort on the lake. Contestants were usually treated to a Coca-Cola party by the previous year's winner. (Marshall County Archives.)

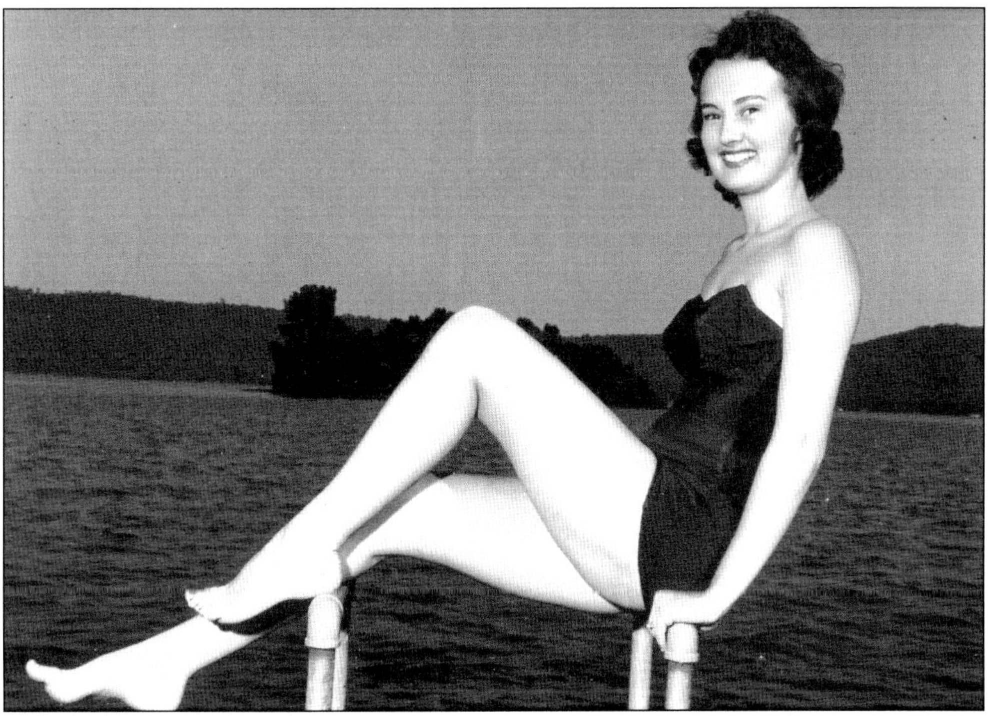

Mary "Prissy" Dunson of Guntersville poses for a photograph while participating in the 1957 Miss Guntersville Lake pageant. Among the other Guntersville contestants were Patricia Patterson, Kathy Thrasher, Oma Jane Rogers, Kitty St. John, Billie Jean Barnard, Angel Wisener, Sally Scott, Mary Virginia Alred, Sandra Shields, "Little" Elsie Crain, Sara Glenn Barnett, Sue Jones, Katy Ward, Carol York, and Sonja Campbell. (Marshall County Archives.)

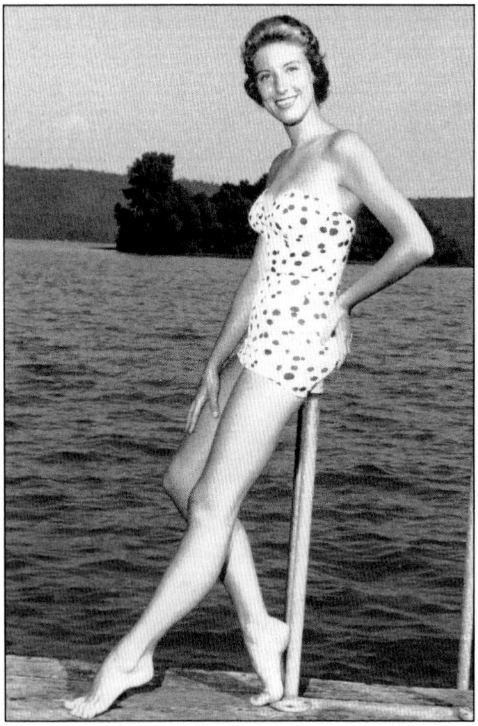

Shown is Katherine "Kitty" Ann St. John, a contestant in the Miss Guntersville Lake pageant of 1957. The pageant that year earned a profit of $1,300 thanks to a combination of entry fees and admission tickets to both the pageant and the accompanying dance. This success did not pale too much with the boat race profit, roughly $2,000. (Marshall County Archives.)

From left to right are Dorothy Jo Oaks, Frances Wells, Angel Wisener, and two unidentified contestants in a Miss Guntersville Lake pageant. The daughter of Dovard and Maxine Oaks, Dorothy Jo graduated from Marshall County High School in 1959 and went to Jacksonville State University. There she was chosen Gem of the Hills in 1960. (Marshall County Archives.)

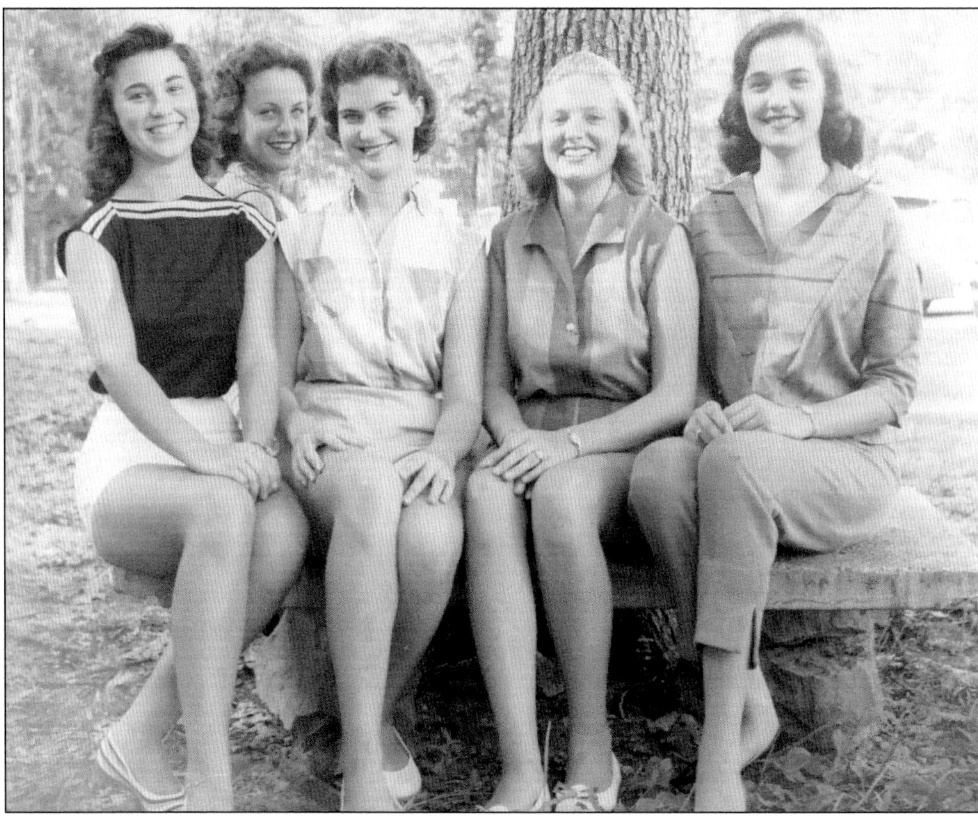

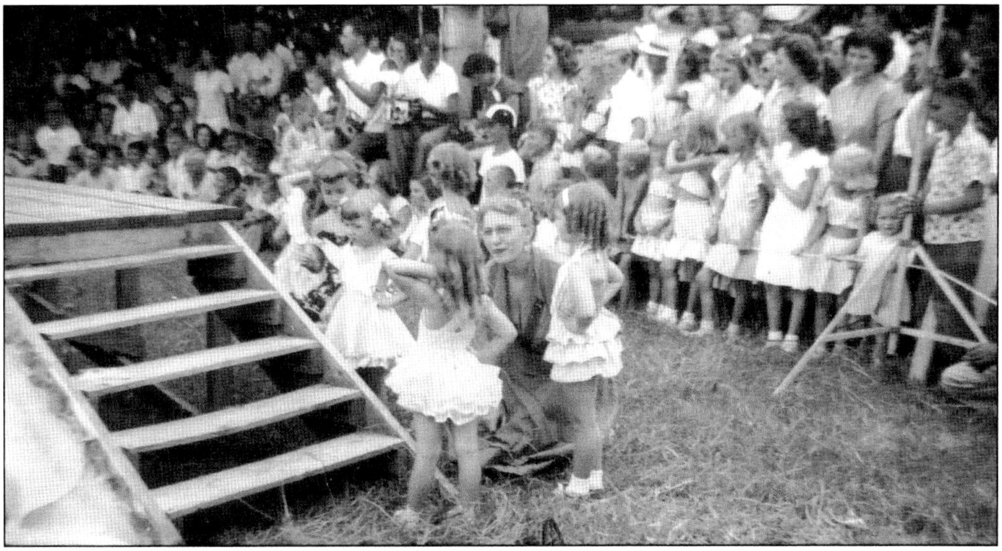

The kneeling woman is Katherine McKinstry Duncan, chair of the Little Miss Guntersville Lake pageant in 1957. She coauthored *The History of Marshall County* with Larry Smith. At one point, she wrote two columns, Chatter and Yesteryears, for the local newspaper, the *Advertiser-Gleam*. According to Smith, "She received numerous awards for her humanitarian contributions." (Marshall County Archives.)

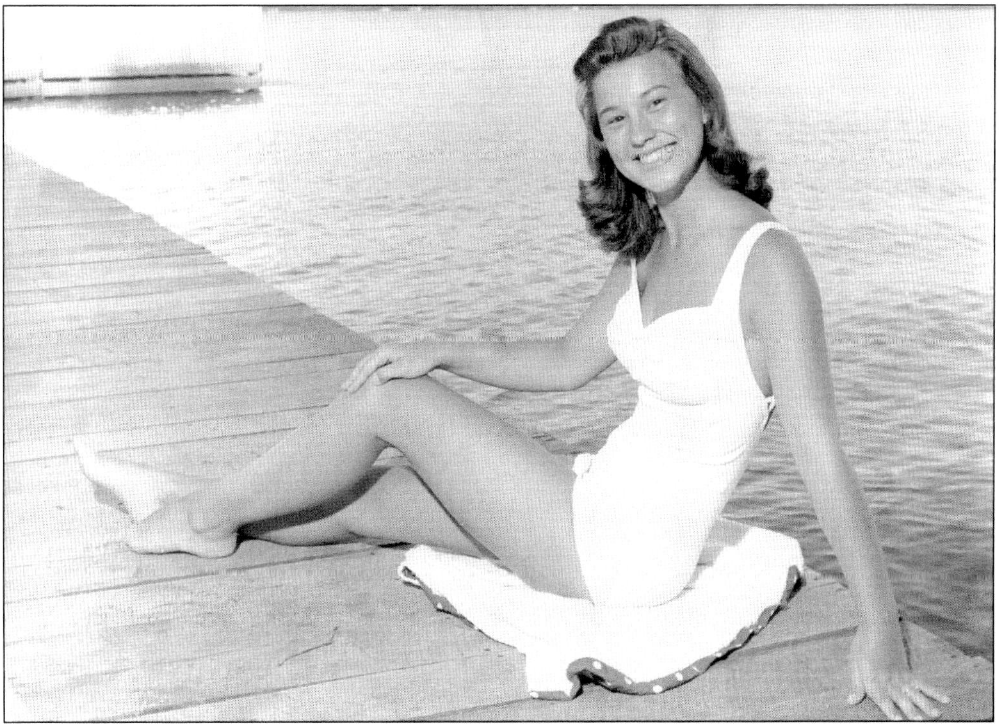

Pictured is Dorothy Jo Oaks, third-place winner in the 1957 Miss Guntersville Lake pageant. That year, the boat races included the four main national championships. Boat race chairmen Hootie Woodall, Bob Bishop Jr., and Charlie Pass were thrilled with this announcement by the American Power Boat Association. (Marshall County Archives.)

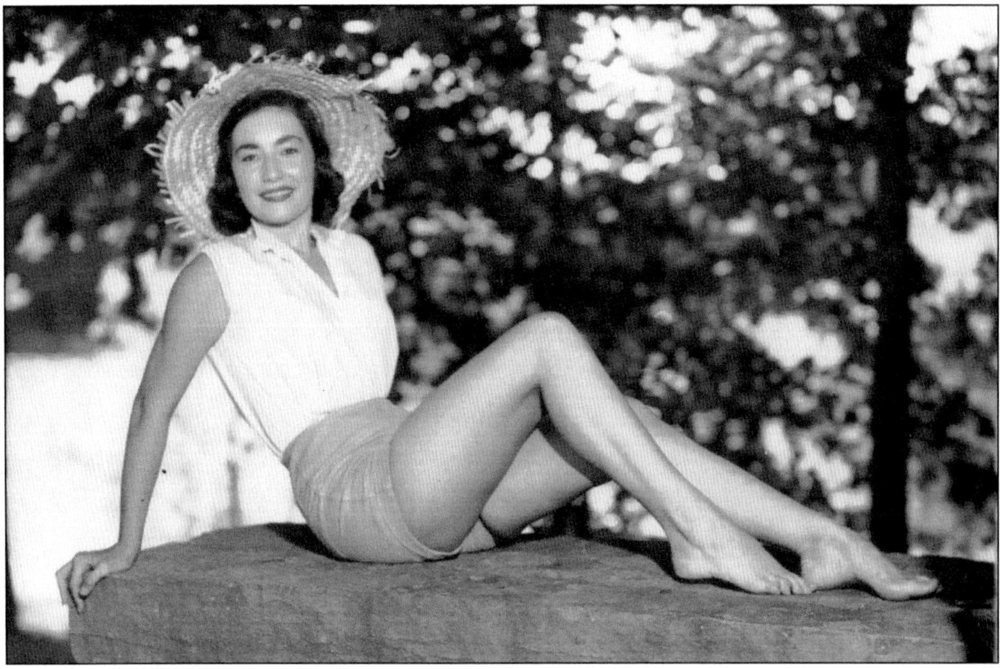

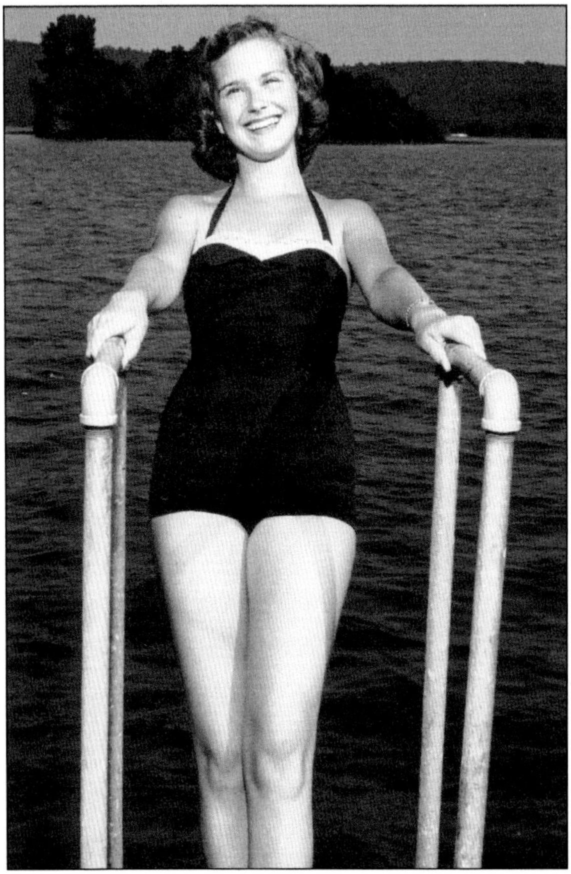

This is Billie Jean Barnard, a contestant in the 1957 and 1958 Miss Guntersville Lake pageants. The daughter of Guntersville residents Henry and Imogene Barnard, Billie Jean attended Marshall County High School, and in addition to belonging to the Beta Club and yearbook staff, she participated in plays and served as a cheerleader. (Marshall County Archives.)

Mary Ruth Manning (shown here) of Guntersville placed second in the 1958 Miss Guntersville Lake pageant. The daughter of Clem and Freelon Manning, Mary Ruth was an alternate in the 1958 County Junior Maid of Cotton pageant, was voted Marshall County High School Miss Sweetheart, and was a runner-up in the Miss Slick Chick contest in Albertville. (Marshall County Archives.)

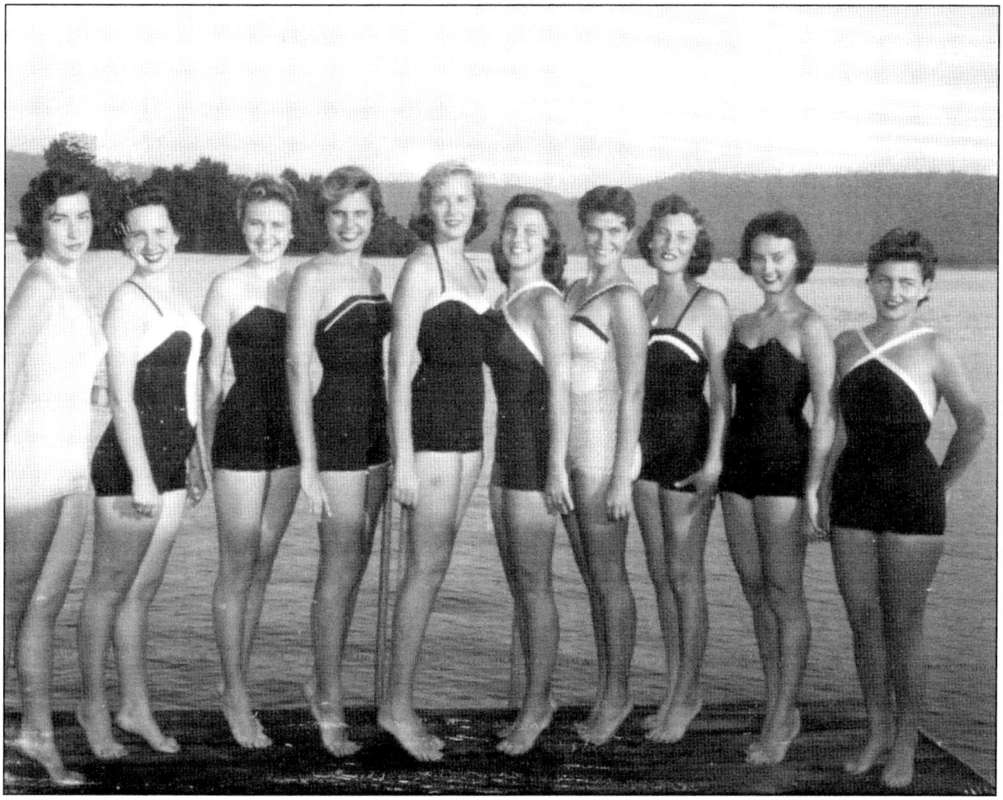

From left to right around 1958 are Miss Guntersville Lake contestants Billie Jean Barnard, Sally Scott, Oma Jane Rogers, Kathy Thrasher, Mary Ruth Manning, Dorothy Jo Oaks, Angel Wisener, Barbara Smith, Prissy Dunson, and Patricia Patterson. Ed Crabtree, chair of the pageant, said, "We believe that this is Alabama's No. 2 annual beauty contest, second only to the Miss Alabama event." (Guntersville Historical Society.)

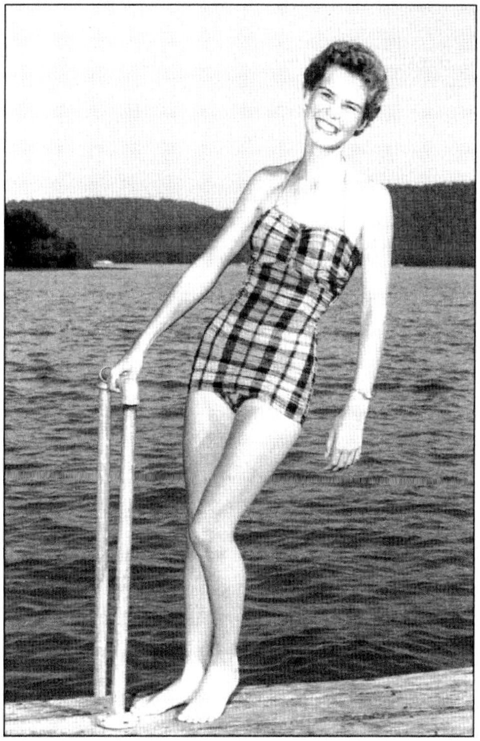

Sandra Shields (shown here) was a contestant in the 1958 Miss Guntersville Lake pageant. The winner that year was Sandra Parsley of Huntsville. Reba Woolley of Meridianville won third place, and Bettye Brooks of Union Grove won fourth place. The judges were Bruno Manz (Huntsville physicist), Helmut Bauer (Huntsville researcher), Gene Parsons (Gadsden architect), and Peggy Elder (Miss Alabama 1947). (Marshall County Archives.)

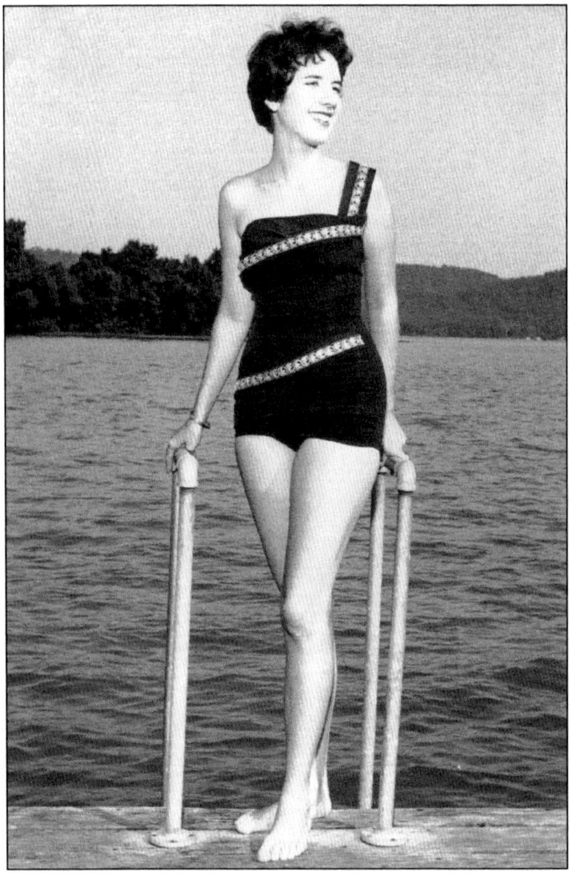

Pictured is Celia Norris Martin, a contestant in the 1958 Miss Guntersville Lake pageant. Of note, 56 girls participated in the Little Miss Guntersville Lake contest that year, and the winners were Elaine Clark of Talladega (first), Rhonda Carroll of Lacey Springs (second), and Connie Ann Huckaby of Arab (third). (Marshall County Archives.)

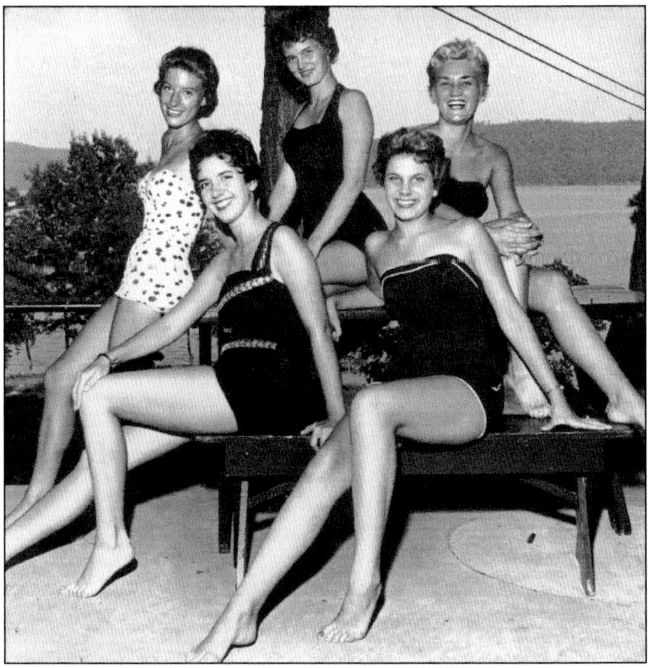

These are Miss Guntersville Lake contestants around 1958. From left to right are (first row) Celia Norris Martin and Kathy Thrasher; (second row) Katherine "Kitty" Ann St. John, Sue Jones, and unidentified. All were from Guntersville. (Marshall County Archives.)

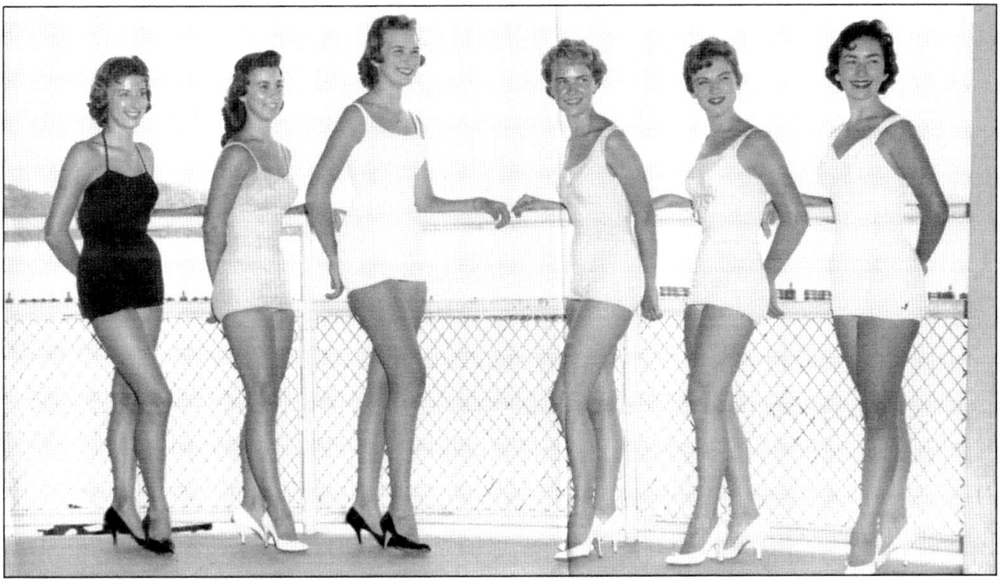

From left to right are Miss Guntersville Lake contestants Katherine "Kitty" Ann St. John, Dorothy Jo Oaks, Mary Ruth Manning, Nell Dunn, Diane Richter, and Billie Jean Barnard. The number of contestants in the Miss Guntersville Lake pageant continued to increase over the years, especially when the contest became a qualifier for Miss Alabama as well as Miss Sun Fun. (Marshall County Archives.)

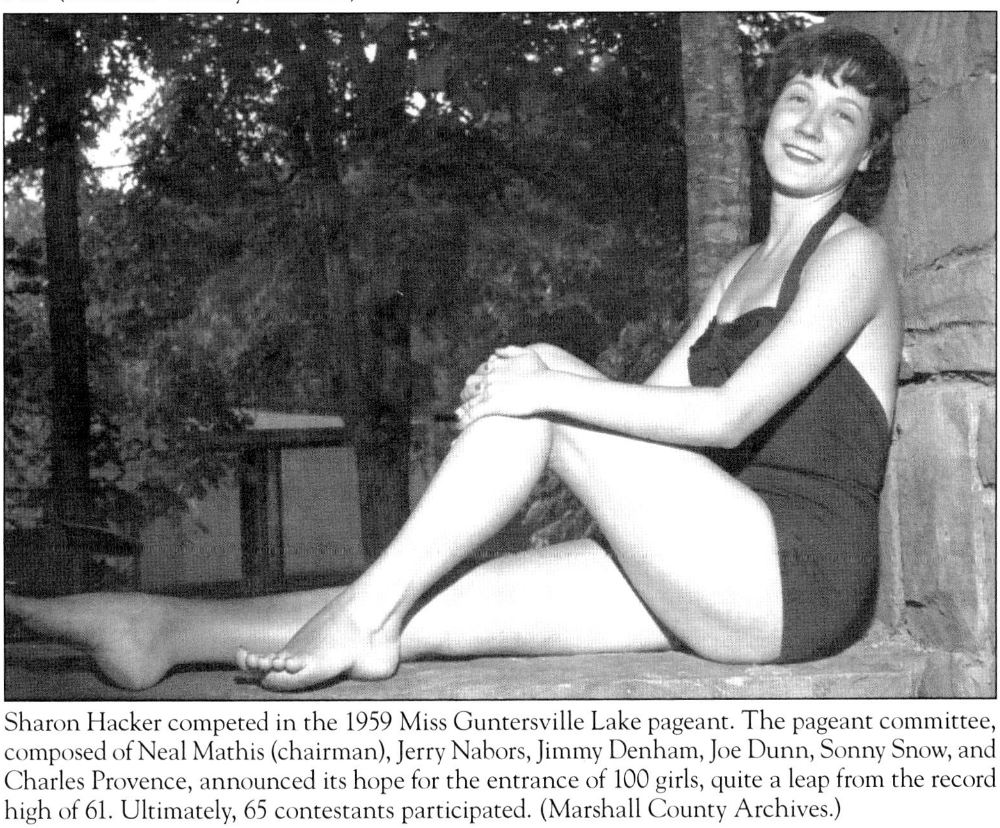

Sharon Hacker competed in the 1959 Miss Guntersville Lake pageant. The pageant committee, composed of Neal Mathis (chairman), Jerry Nabors, Jimmy Denham, Joe Dunn, Sonny Snow, and Charles Provence, announced its hope for the entrance of 100 girls, quite a leap from the record high of 61. Ultimately, 65 contestants participated. (Marshall County Archives.)

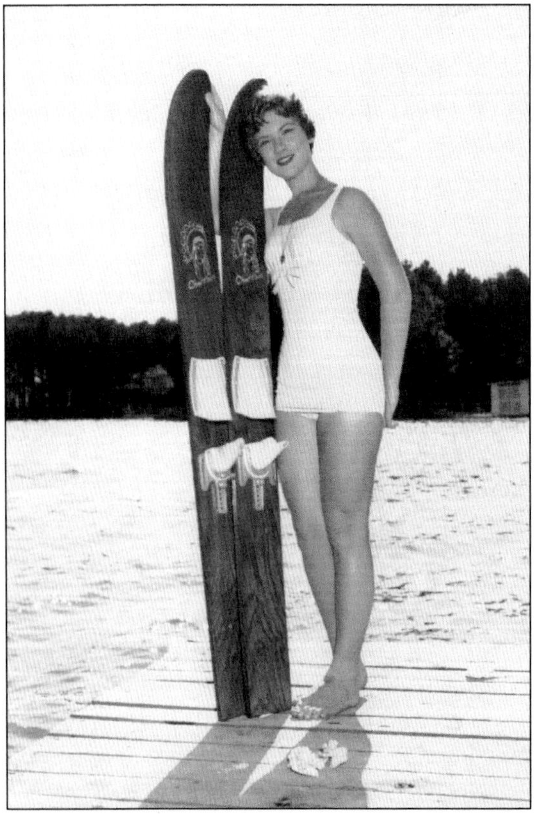

In 1959, Diane Richter (shown here) vied for the title of Miss Guntersville Lake. The winners were Jerolyn Ridgeway of Fort Payne (Miss Guntersville Lake 1959), Jackie Hamilton of Cullman (second), and Martha Campbell of Scottsboro (third). The winner of the Little Miss Guntersville Lake pageant was Andrea McInnis of Arab. (Marshall County Archives.)

These are 1960 Miss Guntersville Lake contestants. From left to right are Frances Silvey (Arab), Mary Sue Bodine (Arab), Mary Dudley Call (Cullman), Carol Goodlett (Cullman), Patti Patrick (Cullman), Deeanna Kirby (Arab), and Melissa Folsom (Cullman). Melissa is the daughter of former Alabama governor James "Big Jim" Folsom. (Marshall County Archives.)

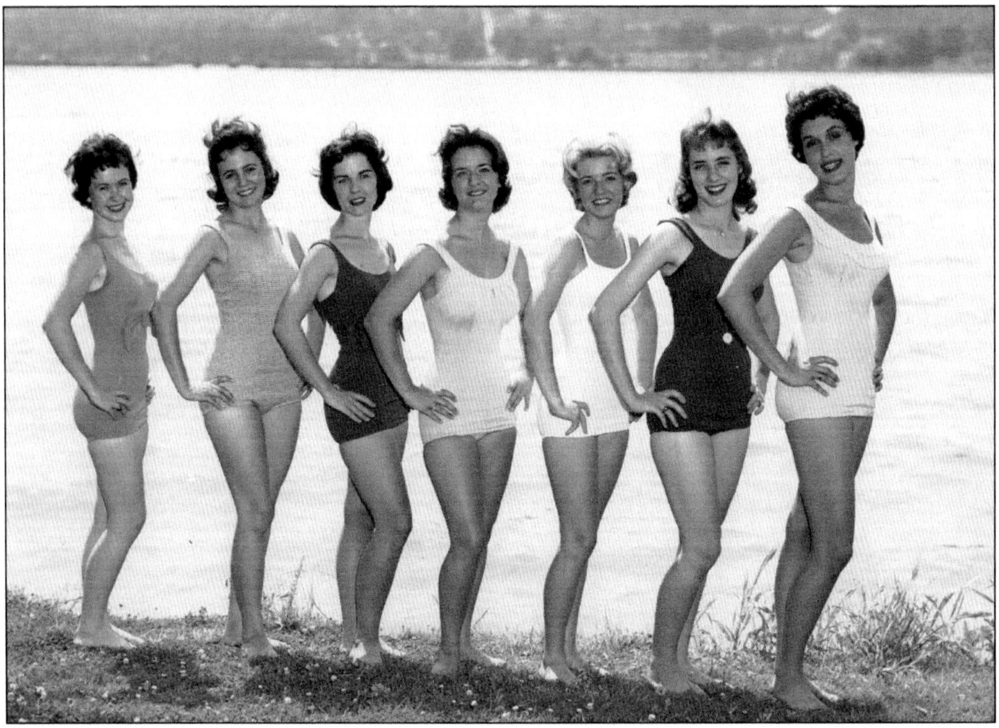

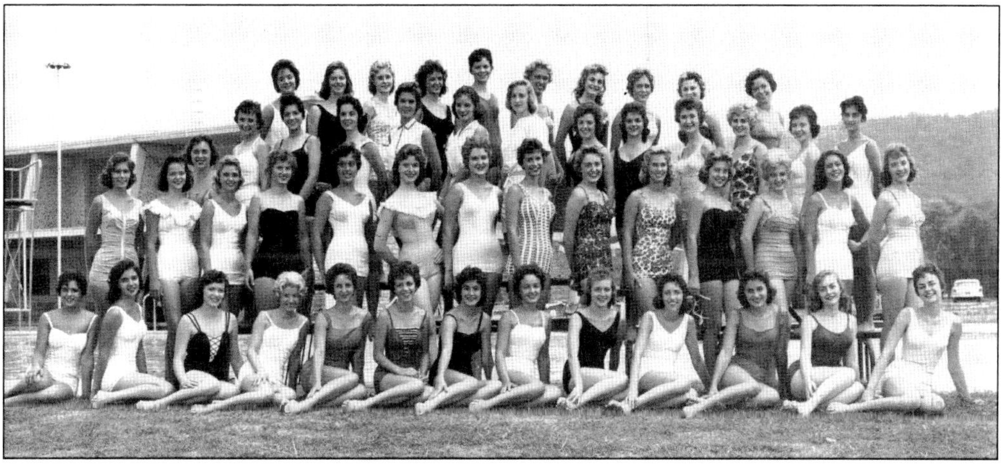

In 1960, wind, rain, and lightning caused the crowds to flee for shelter during the boat races. The sudden storm damaged the concession booths and judges' stand. The downpour soaked Harla Briggs (Miss Guntersville Lake 1960) and her court. When the spectators reassembled, the Jaycees had no way to determine who had paid, so latecomers received free admission. (Marshall County Archives.)

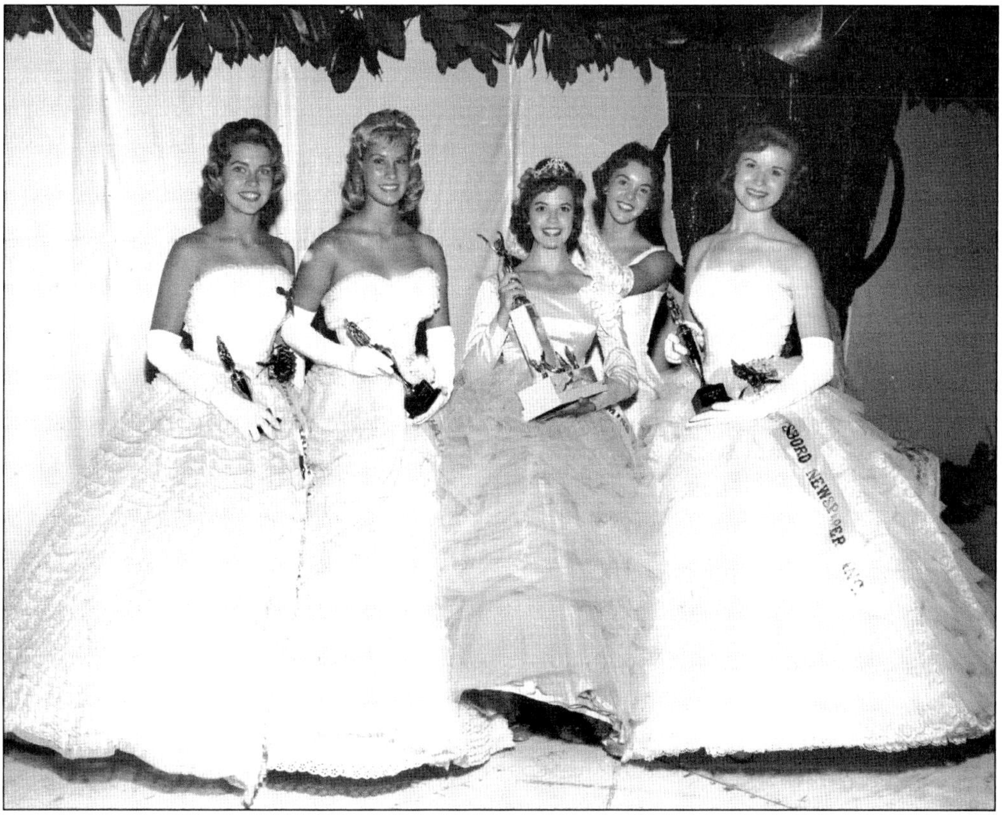

From left to right are Katherine Pugh of Huntsville (fourth), Ginger Poitevint of Huntsville (third), Harla Briggs of Birmingham (Miss Guntersville Lake 1960), Jerolyn Ridgeway of Fort Payne (Miss Guntersville Lake 1959), and Martha Campbell of Scottsboro (second). Poitevint was later crowned Miss Sun Fun at Myrtle Beach in 1963. (Marshall County Archives.)

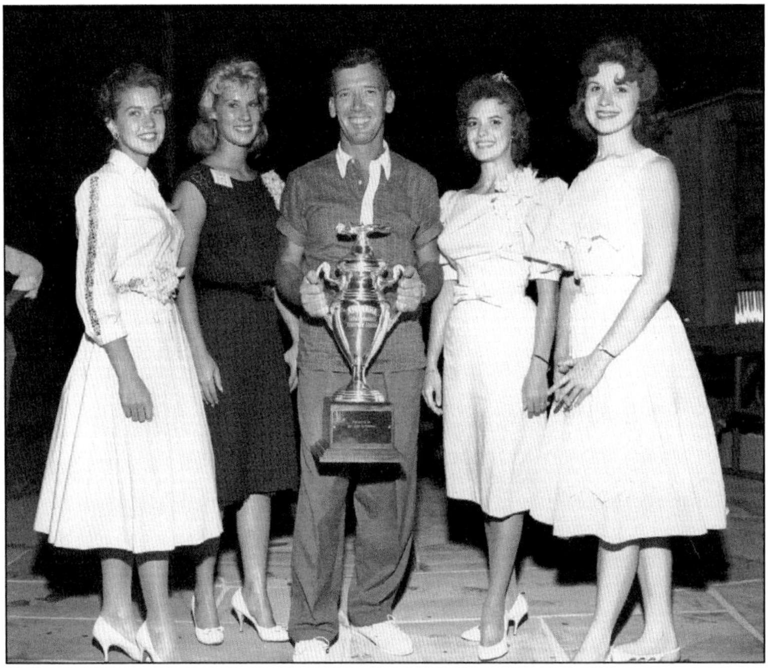

From left to right are Katherine Pugh (fourth), Ginger Poitevint (third), Enas "Ennie" Argence of New Orleans, Harla Briggs (Miss Guntersville Lake 1960), and Martha Campbell (second). On July 30, 1960, the *Advertiser-Gleam* reported that Argent and his boat *Gun Shy* won "both heats in the 266-cubic-inch class." He also won the Governor's Trophy. (Marshall County Archives.)

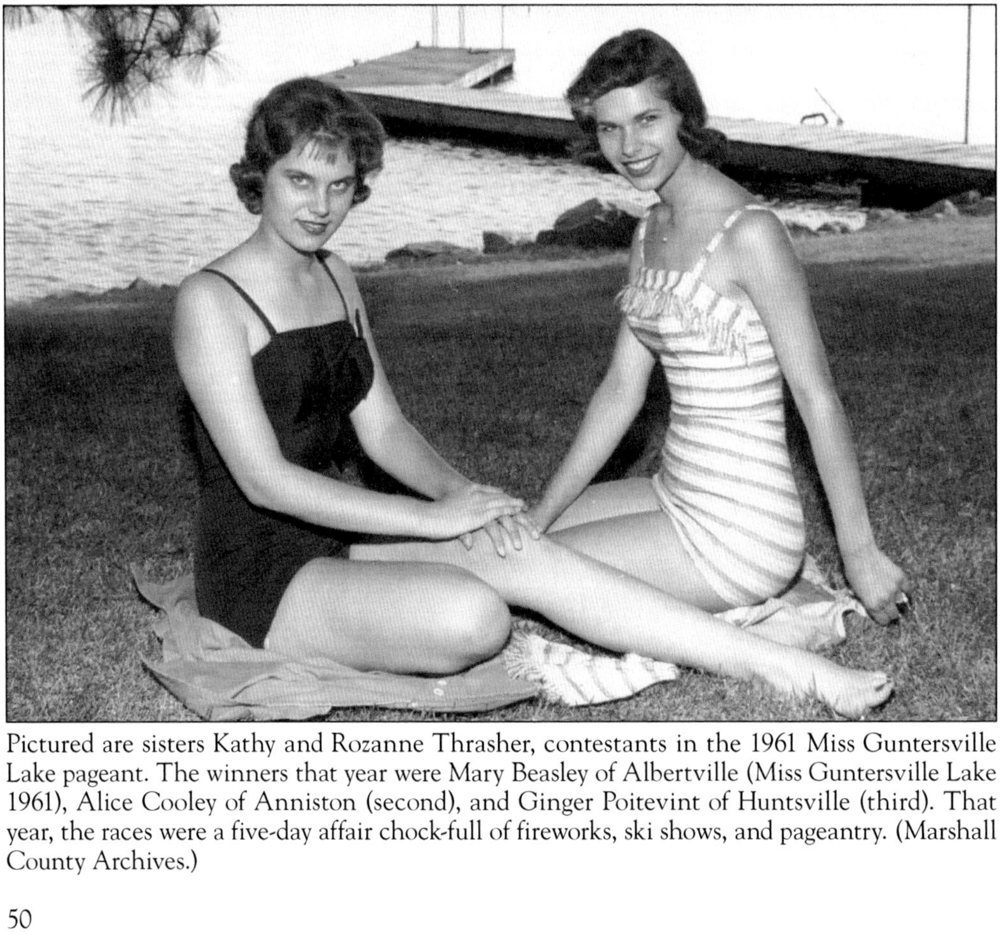

Pictured are sisters Kathy and Rozanne Thrasher, contestants in the 1961 Miss Guntersville Lake pageant. The winners that year were Mary Beasley of Albertville (Miss Guntersville Lake 1961), Alice Cooley of Anniston (second), and Ginger Poitevint of Huntsville (third). That year, the races were a five-day affair chock-full of fireworks, ski shows, and pageantry. (Marshall County Archives.)

Posing is Haleyville's Sandra Howell (Miss Guntersville Lake 1962). The other winners were Mary Hamilton of Athens (second), Martha Yancey of Altoona (third), Sherry Douglas of Guntersville (Miss Congeniality), and Lynn Hawkins of Mobile (Miss Photogenic). The winners of the 1962 Little Miss Guntersville Lake contest were Pam Godfrey of Madison (first), Mary Lowden of Albertville (second), and Elizabeth Isdell of Guntersville (third). (Guntersville Museum.)

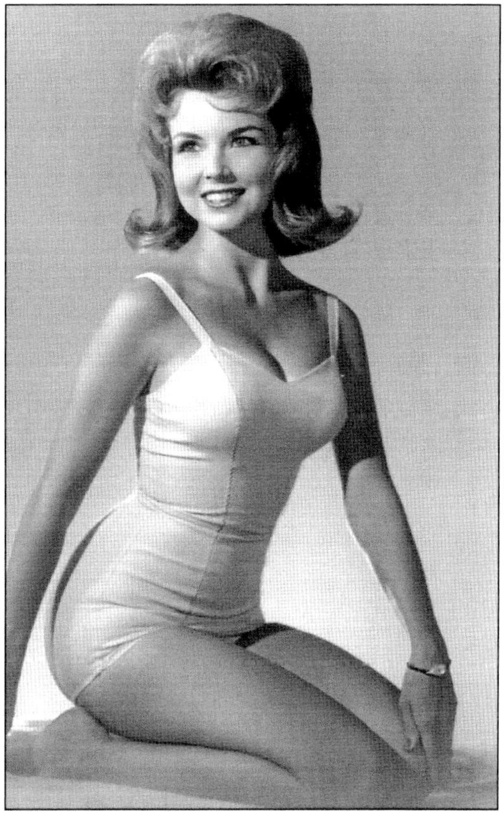

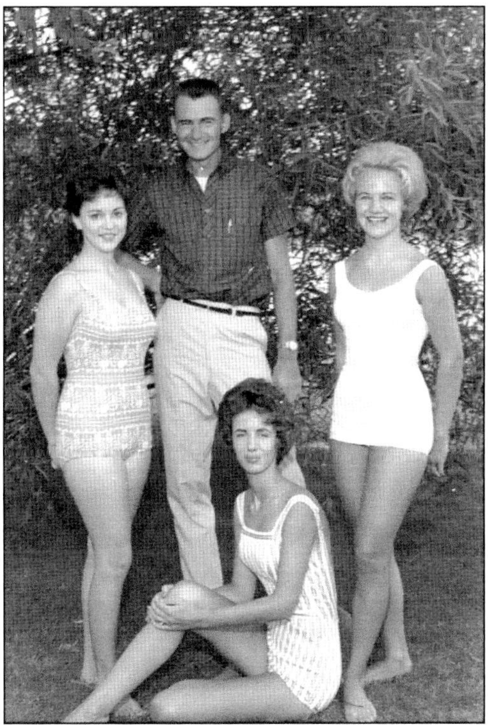

From left to right are 1962 Miss Guntersville Lake contestants Gloria Wright (Point of Pines), Doris Chafin (Union Grove), and Sherry Douglas (Beech Creek) with Bob Rice, chair of the pageant committee. Sherry Douglas became homecoming queen of Marshall County High School in 1963. (Marshall County Archives.)

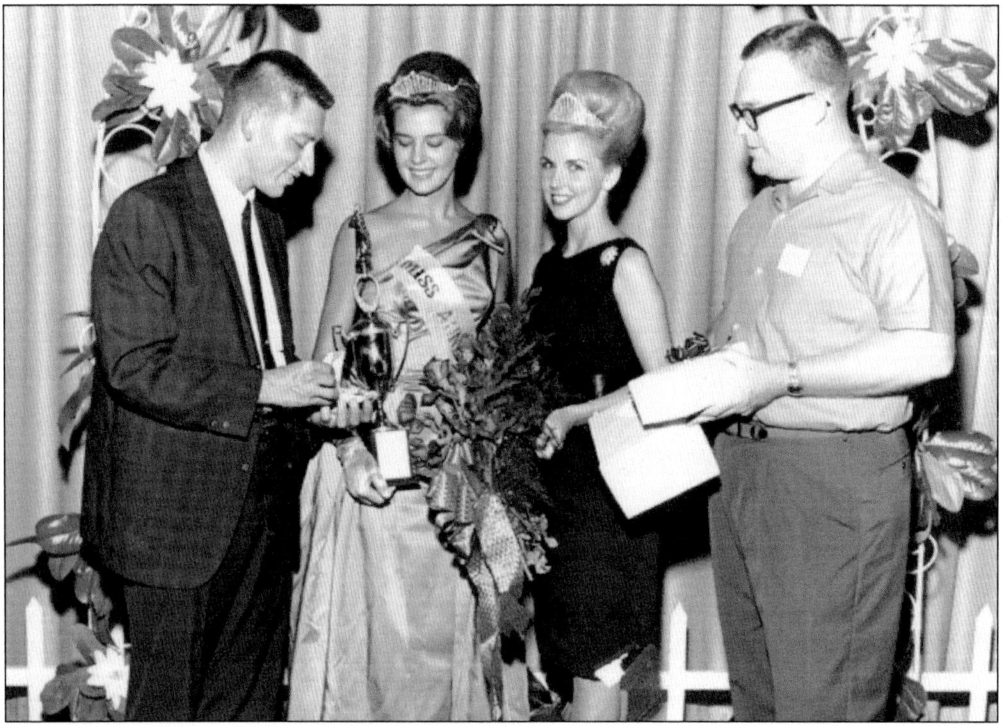

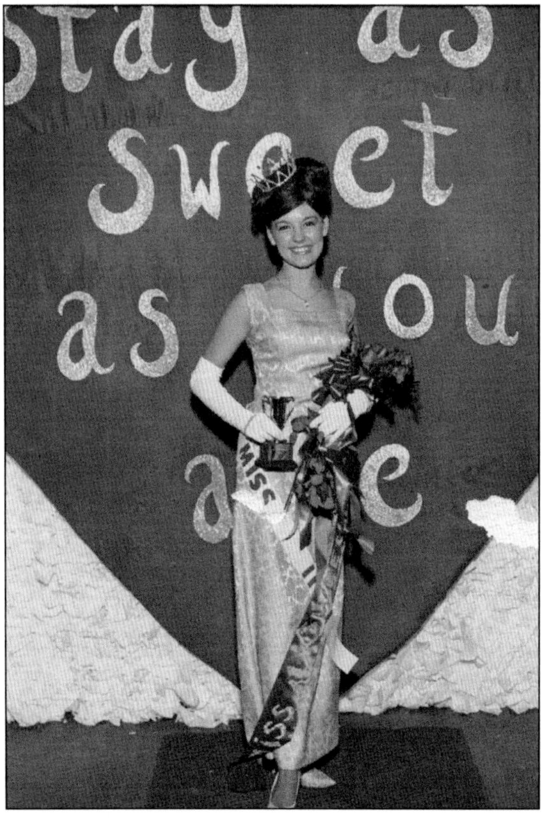

From left to right are Tommy Campbell, Linda Vaughn of Anniston (Miss Guntersville Lake 1963), Sandra Howell (Miss Guntersville Lake 1962), and Ed Crabtree (Jaycee president). Other girls honored that night were Kathy Miller of Mobile (second), Sandra Hubbard of Gadsden, and Manola Harper of Fyffe. Vaughn became Miss Sun Fun USA in 1964. (Guntersville Museum.)

Barbara Emmenegger (shown) was selected Miss Sweetheart of Marshall County High School in 1966. Cindy Emmenegger and Lucy Hallman won second and third place, respectively. For the first time since the pageant's beginning in 1952, the top two places went to sisters. Barbara was crowned by Janette Kelly, who won second place in 1965. (Guntersville Museum.)

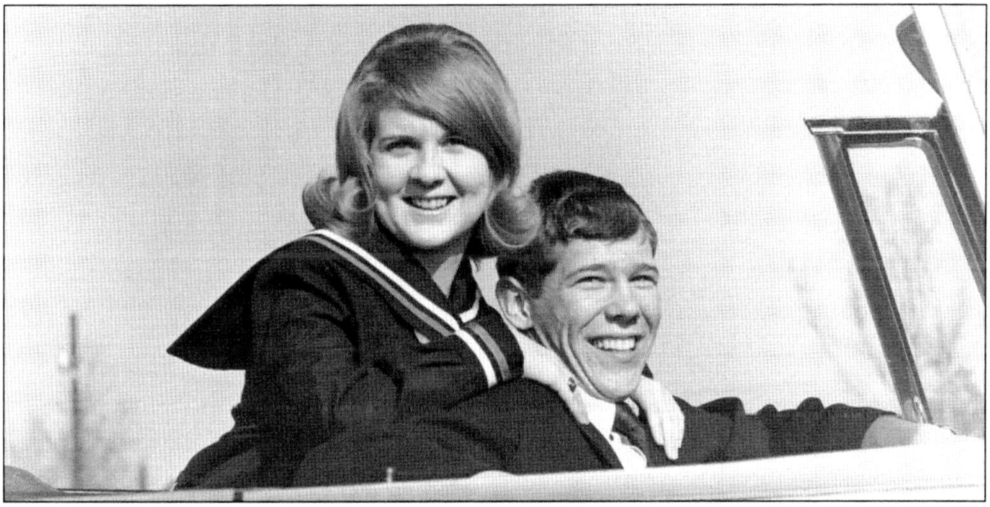

Shown are Nancy Gross (Miss Sweetheart of Marshall County High School 1963) and Tommy Ross. The daughter of Ruth and Welch Gross, Nancy moved to Los Angeles and worked as a publicist specializing in the entertainment industry. Her late husband, John Hill, was an Emmy-winning television and movie writer. Nancy currently lives in Las Vegas. (Guntersville Museum.)

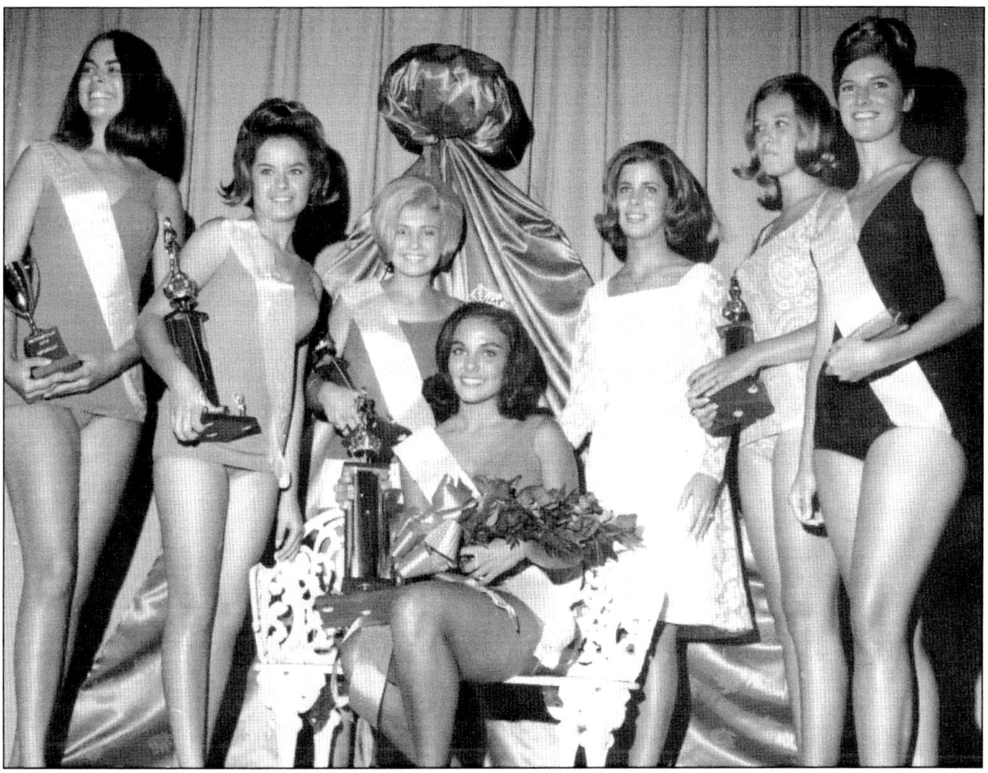

Seated is Rebecca Dyar of Arab (Miss Guntersville Lake 1967). Standing, from left to right, are Mary Hughes Somerville of Aliceville (Miss Congeniality), Pamela Jo Wright of Huntsville (second), Pamela Locklear of Guntersville (third), Sharon Herman (Miss Guntersville Lake 1966), Bobbie Nix of Huntsville (fourth), and Gail Smith of Pulaski, Tennessee (Miss Photogenic). Dyar was also chosen Miss Arab in 1964. (Gail Smith Ingrum.)

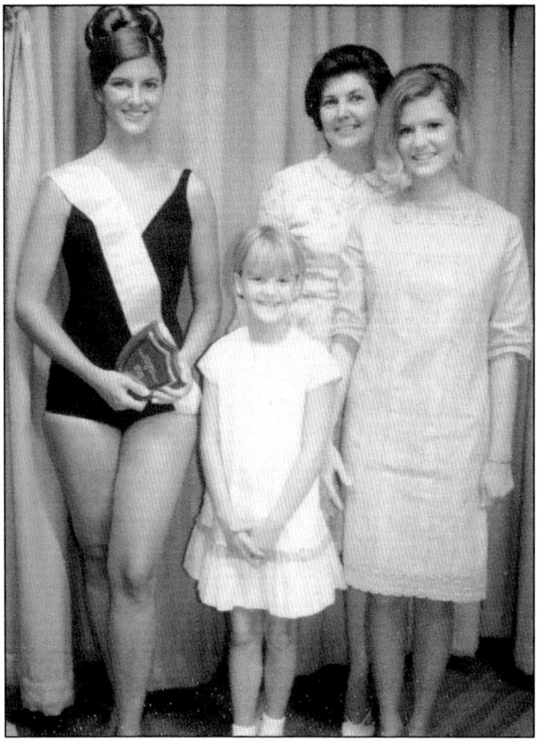

Gail Smith (far left) won Miss Photogenic in the 1967 Miss Guntersville Lake pageant. The others, from left to right, are her sister Dee Ann Smith; her mother, Ida Will Willis Smith (Miss Guntersville Lake 1946); and Gail's other sister Ginny Smith. Gail continues to be a frequent visitor to Guntersville. (Gail Smith Ingrum.)

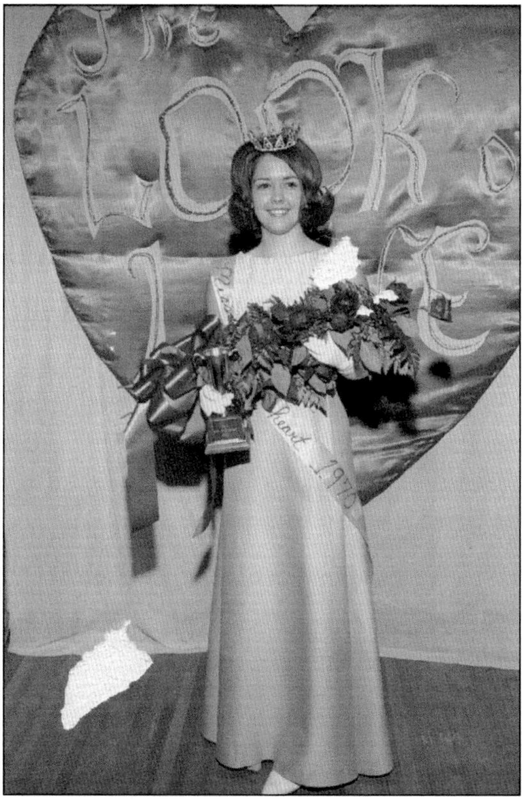

Pictured here, Kathy Smith (Miss Sweetheart 1970) was crowned by Debbie Kennedy, the 1969 winner. Alternates were Theresa Stone (second), Renee Brooks (third), and Belinda Conley (fourth). Others in the top 10 were Debbie Hamric, Yonnie Williams, Mavis Lyles, Vickie Morgan, Cathy Hardin, and Carol Rauschenberg. (Guntersville Museum.)

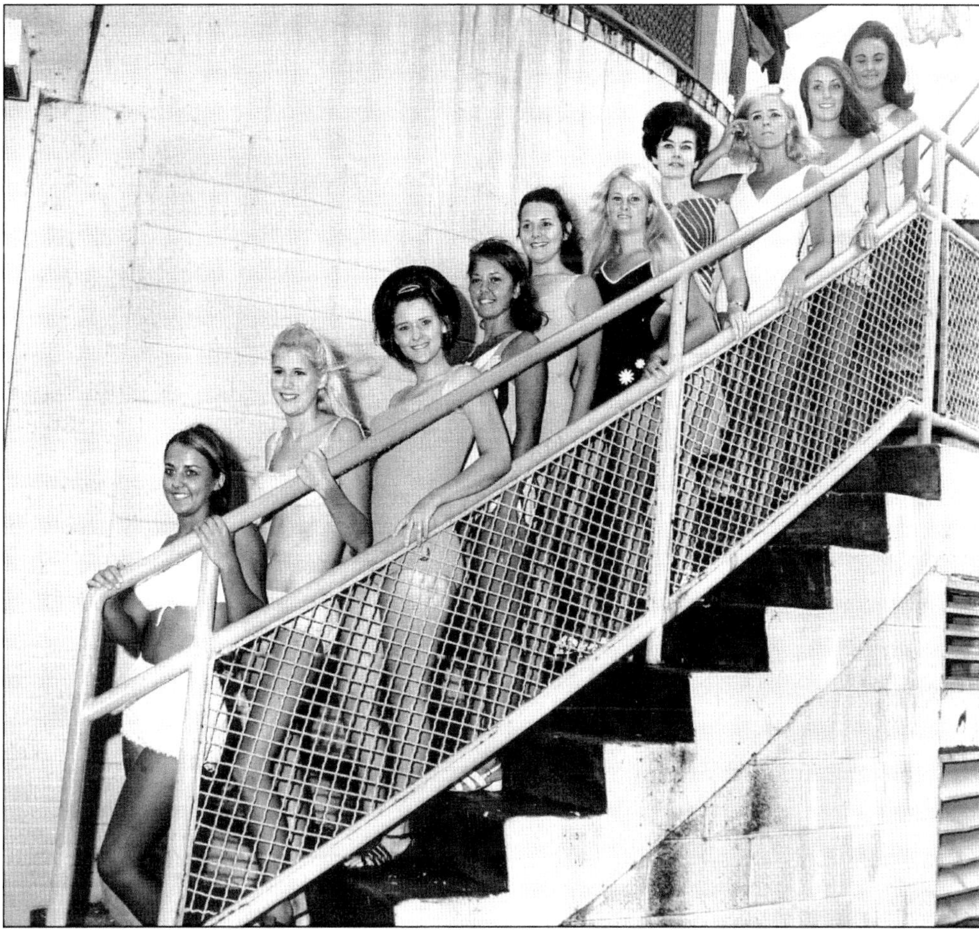

From left to right are contestants in the 1970 Miss Guntersville Lake pageant: Vickie Morgan (Guntersville), Becky Clay (Guntersville), Vicki Gibson (Union Grove), Kathy Smith (Guntersville), Patty Shumate (Arab), Adonis Hubble (Guntersville), Jane Sport (Guntersville), Marsha Johnson (Albertville), Kathy Black (Arab), and Martha Dyar (Arab). (Marshall County Archives.)

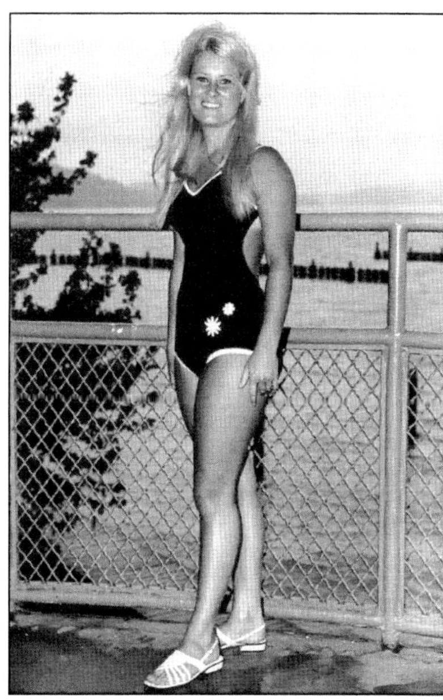

This is Adonis Hubble of Guntersville, a contestant in the 1970 Miss Guntersville Lake pageant. Between 1970 and 1974, the winners were as follows: Caron Halsey of Anniston (1970), Justine Mannes of Alexander City (1971), Kathie McDaniel of Alexander City (1972), Debra Walters of Gardendale (1973), and Becky Hallman of Guntersville (1974). (Marshall County Archives.)

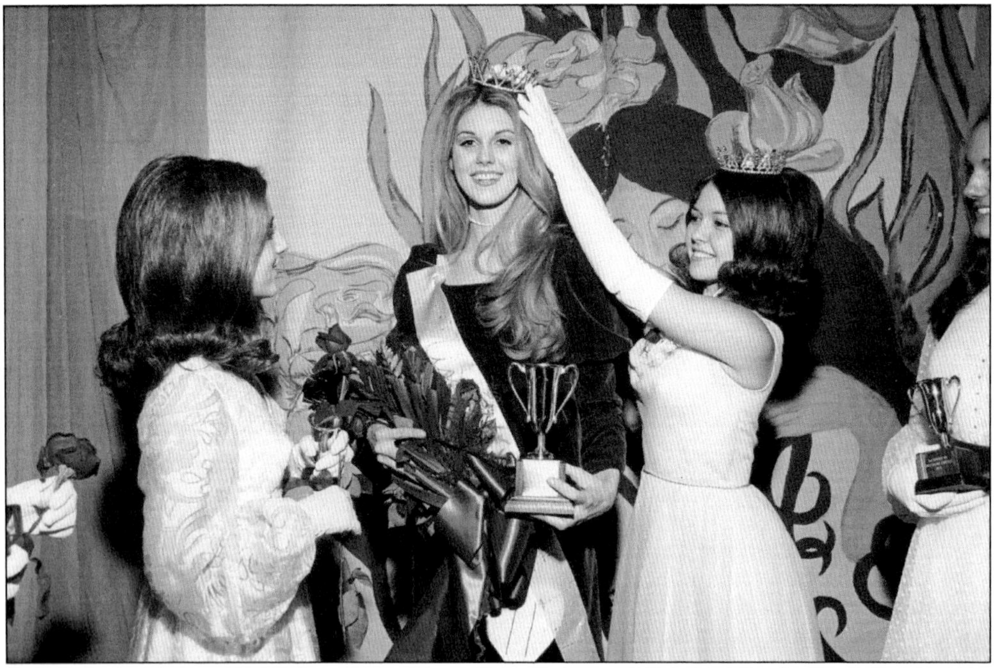

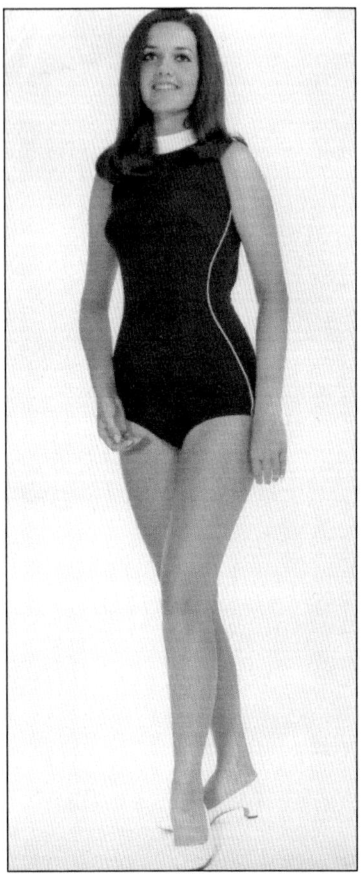

From left to right are Rita Wright (second), Gwen Deck (Miss Sweetheart 1971), Kathy Smith (Miss Sweetheart 1970), and Lisa Dorman (third). Not pictured is Marianne Pockstaller (fourth). Eighty-one girls competed, and among the top 10 were Renee Brooks, Sherry LeCroy, Kathy Bucher, Bonita Hubble, Martha Jean Dyar, and Gina Emmenegger. (Guntersville Museum.)

This is Kathie McDaniel (Miss Guntersville Lake 1972). At the time, she was majoring in business at the University of Alabama. Second and third place that year went to Connie Morgan and Paula Entrekin. The winner of the Little Miss Guntersville Lake pageant was Lori Ann Dunn of Guntersville. (Guntersville Museum.)

These are the members of 1974 Miss Sweetheart court shown with flowers and trophies. From left to right are Valina Reynolds, Annette Todd (Miss Sweetheart 1974), Meg Whitmire, and Marianne Pockstaller. In the top 10 were Sheila Matthews, Nancy Boggus, Teresa Grayson, Kathy Cornelius, Rita Jones, and Lisa Dorman. (Guntersville Museum.)

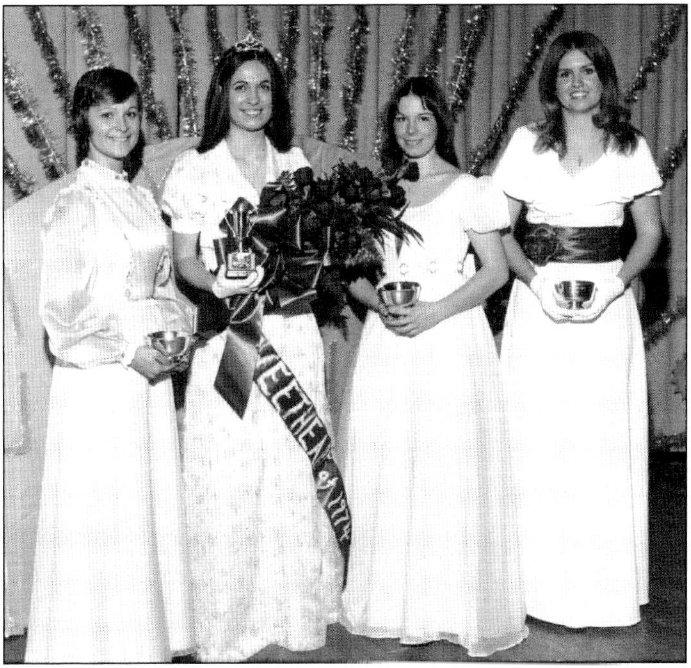

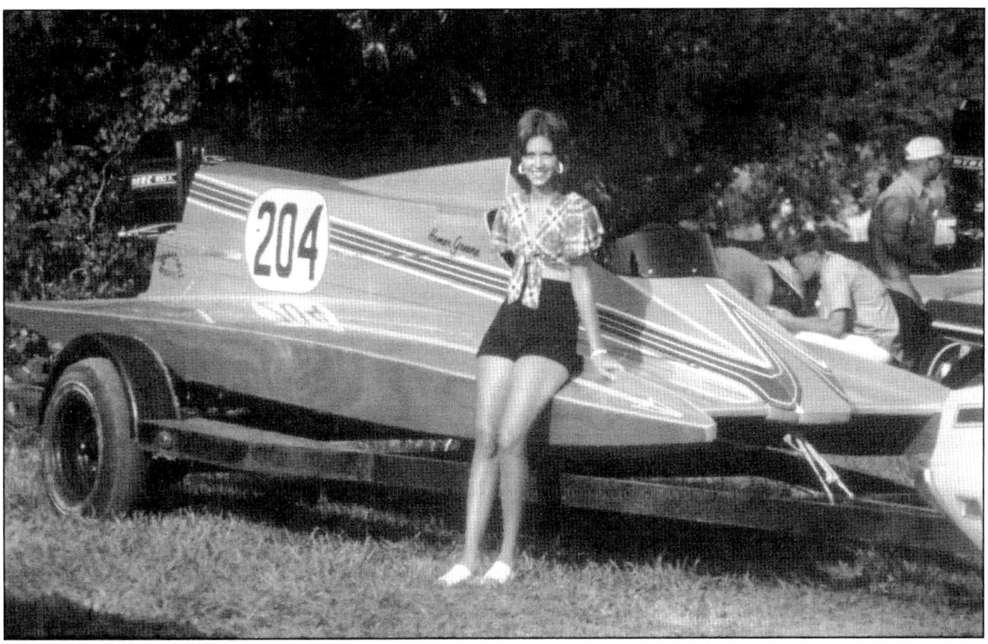

Pictured is Arab's Amanda Gibbs (Miss Guntersville Lake 1975). The second- and third-place winners were Myra Pledger of Horton and Velinda Hawkins of Arab. Between 1976 and 1980, the winners were Ginger Howard (1976), Renae Smith (1977), Mitzi Gutierrez (1978), Sherry Anderton (1979), and Rhonda Handley (1980). All of these girls were from Arab. (Guntersville Museum.)

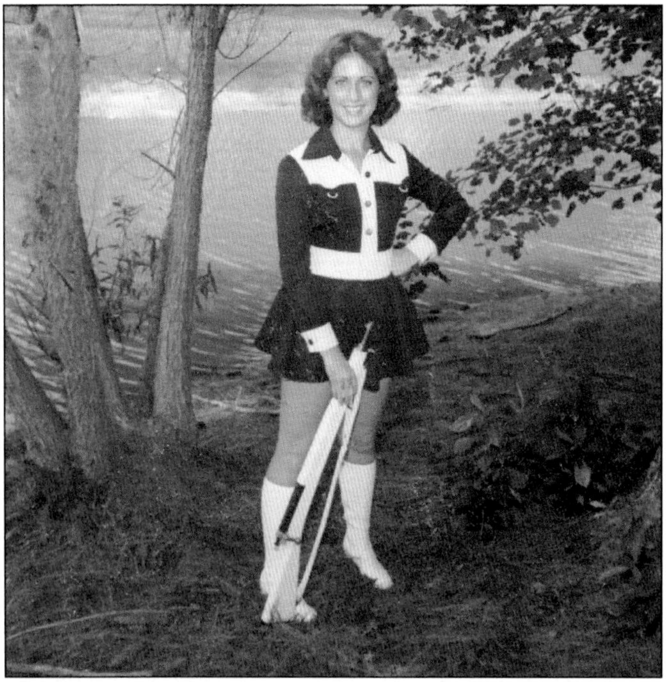

Mary Black (Arab), the daughter of Annette Haislip, was Miss Congeniality in the 1977 Miss Guntersville Lake pageant. That year, the other winners were Renae Smith (Miss Guntersville Lake 1977), Gina Gibbs (second), and Mitzi Gutierrez (third). The winners of the Little Miss Guntersville Lake contest were Lisa Wilson (first), Nikki DeNan Cain (second), and Jill King (third). (Mary Yarber Frank.)

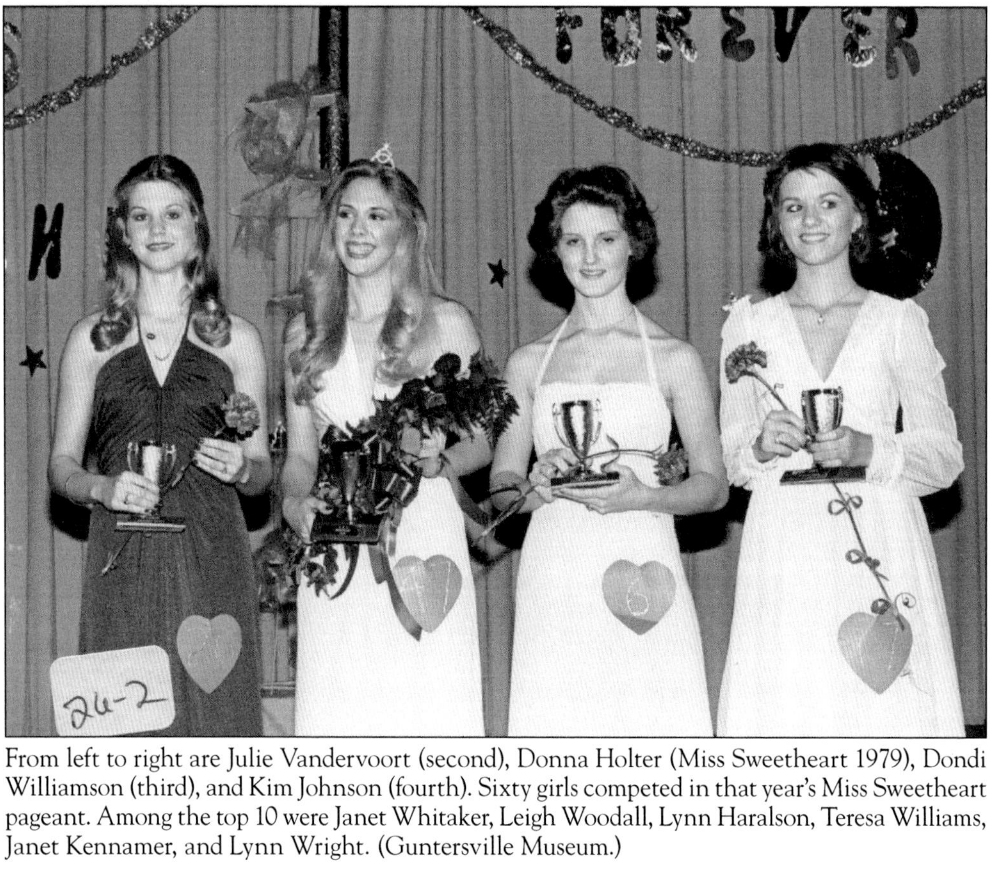

From left to right are Julie Vandervoort (second), Donna Holter (Miss Sweetheart 1979), Dondi Williamson (third), and Kim Johnson (fourth). Sixty girls competed in that year's Miss Sweetheart pageant. Among the top 10 were Janet Whitaker, Leigh Woodall, Lynn Haralson, Teresa Williams, Janet Kennamer, and Lynn Wright. (Guntersville Museum.)

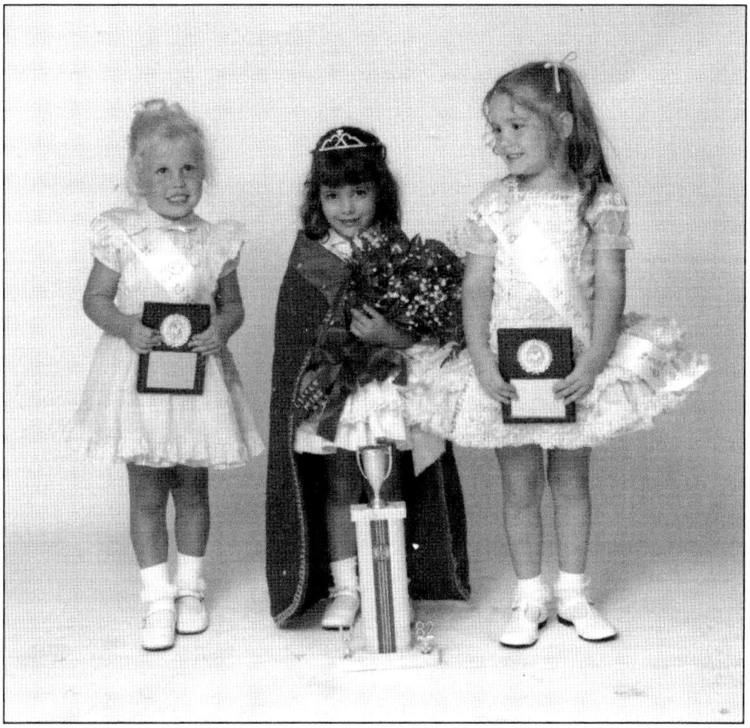

From left to right are the 1982 Little Miss Guntersville Lake winners: Amy Finch (second), Lindsey Couch (first), and Angela Byrd (third). Lindsey, daughter of Rick and Jana Couch, later became a member of Marshall County Youth Leadership, earned a college degree, worked as a teacher, and became a stay-at-home mom. She and her husband, Michael, have three children: Mary Margaret, Harper Jane, and Jack. (Lindsey Couch Douglas.)

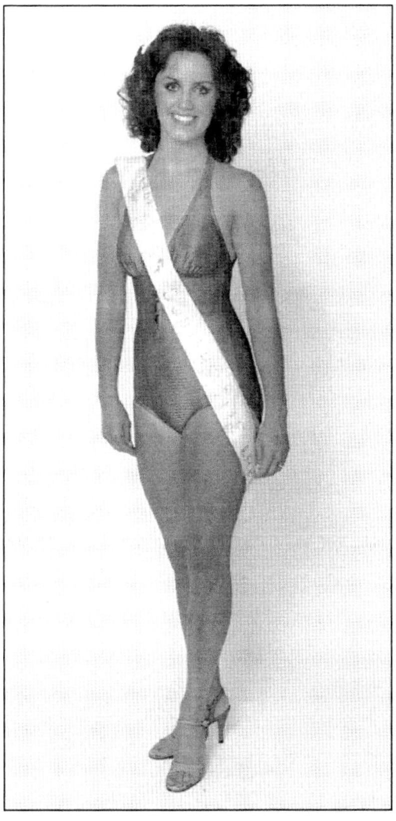

Kim Copeland of Arab (Miss Guntersville Lake 1982), daughter of Teena and Dwight Copeland, was among the youngest winners in the pageant's history. She was also chosen Miss Mid-South at the Mid-South Marching Band Festival at Gadsden that fall. Other Miss Guntersville Lake winners that year were Peggy Covington of Arab (second), Rhonda Johnson of Arab (third), and Lori Copeland of Douglas (Miss Congeniality). (Kimberly Copeland Stewart.)

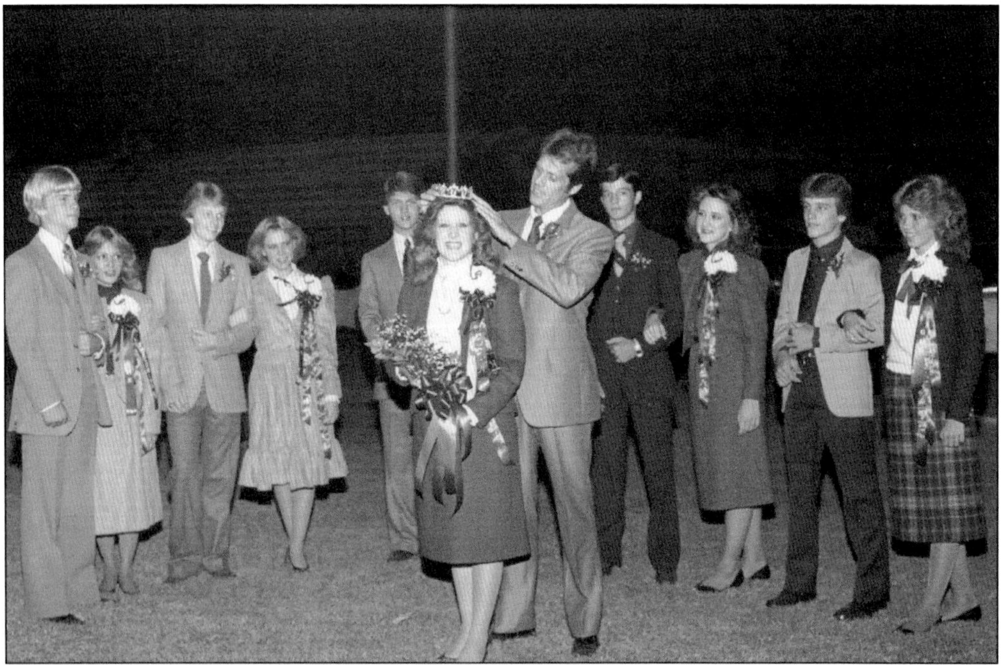

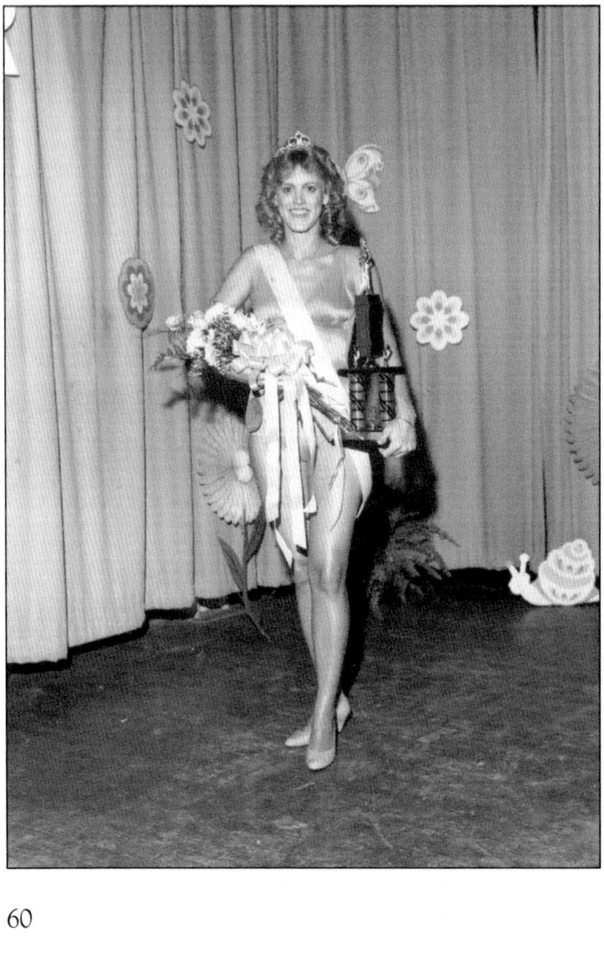

In 1982, Tia Andoe (front) is crowned homecoming queen by Guntersville High School principal Les Click. Attendants are, from left to right, Kim Jerrell (sophomore), Sandy Stone (senior), Kim Andoe (junior), and Julie Brown (freshman). The court was honored by a parade and celebrated in a ceremony during halftime at the football game. The escorts are unidentified. (Guntersville Museum.)

This is Jenny Barnard of Hebron (Miss Guntersville Lake 1983). Christie Hunt and Rhonda Johnson, both of Arab, won second and third place, respectively. Between 1984 and 1986, the winners were Tricia Oliver of Arab (1984); Kimberly Plunkett of Arab (1985); and Anne Marie Wright of Douglas (1986). While pageants were planned for the remainder of the 1980s, each was cancelled due to low participation. (*Advertiser-Gleam.*)

Three

RECREATION AND TOURISM

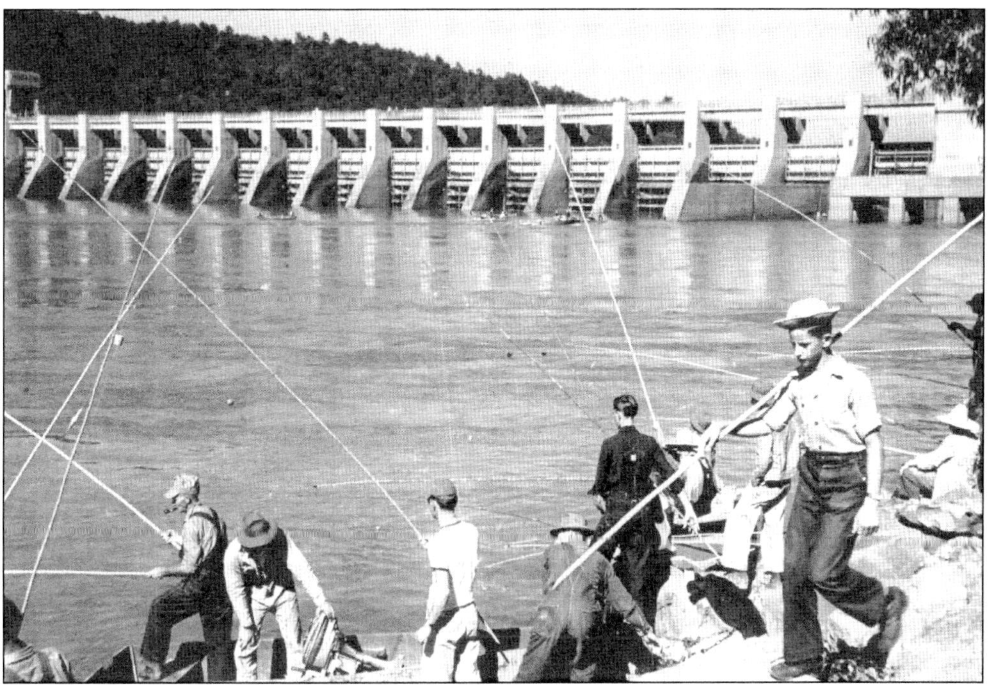

Fishing has always been popular at the Tennessee Valley Authority Guntersville Dam. Standing in boats or at the base of a rock embankment, these men and boys are using cane poles. Many preferred to make their own cane poles, while others purchased them in stores. Fishing with live bait, some preferred no aids, while others used bobbers or bells. (*Advertiser-Gleam.*)

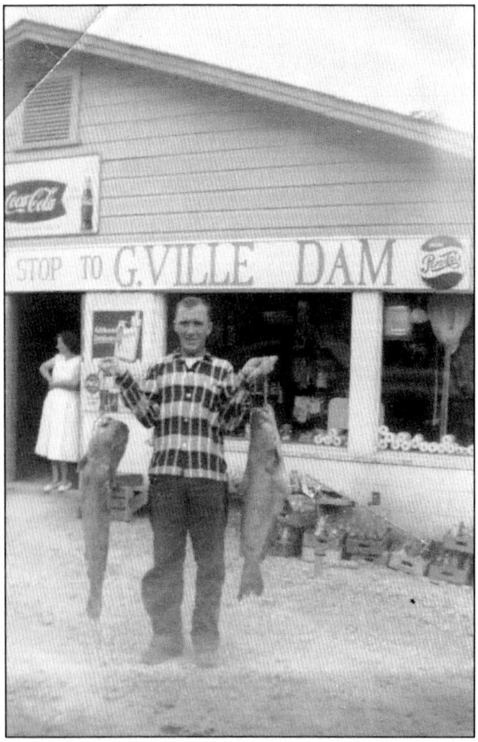

In this c. 1950s image, Donald J. Snow is shown displaying a catch in front of N.P. Brooks's store at the end of Snow Point Road, which leads to the Tennessee Valley Authority Guntersville Dam. Don J. relished angling for crappie, jack salmon (sauger), and especially catfish. When catfishing, his preferred technique was bumping bottom. (Authors' collection.)

A young Quintus "Buddy" Taylor Jr. fishes on Lake Guntersville. The son of Quintus "Dono" and Loree Taylor, he became a professional photographer. His father was elected sheriff in 1932. Over the years, his mother worked at Kate Griffith's dress shop, Hammer's, and Larue Kennamer's Mill End Store. (Buddy Taylor.)

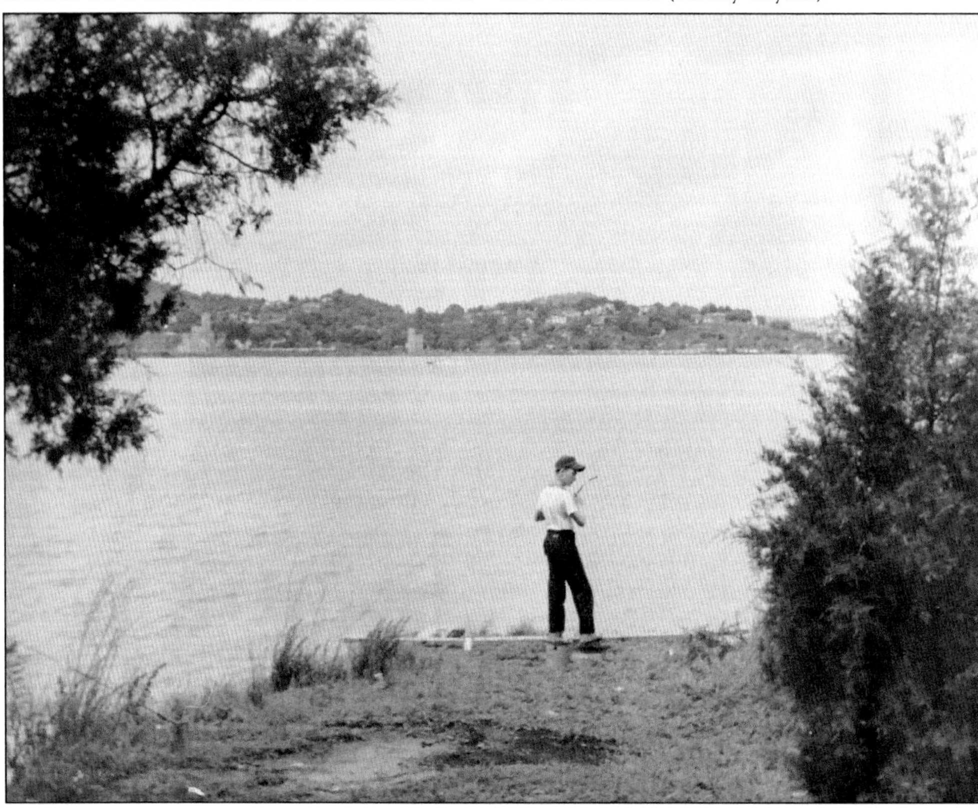

Pictured is John T. Sulzby with a large bass. A vice president of the First National Bank of Guntersville, he was a Mason, a Shriner, and a president of the Civitan Club. He came to the city in 1927 and retired in 1957. According to the *Advertiser-Gleam*, Sulzby fished twice a day year-round. (Marshall County Archives.)

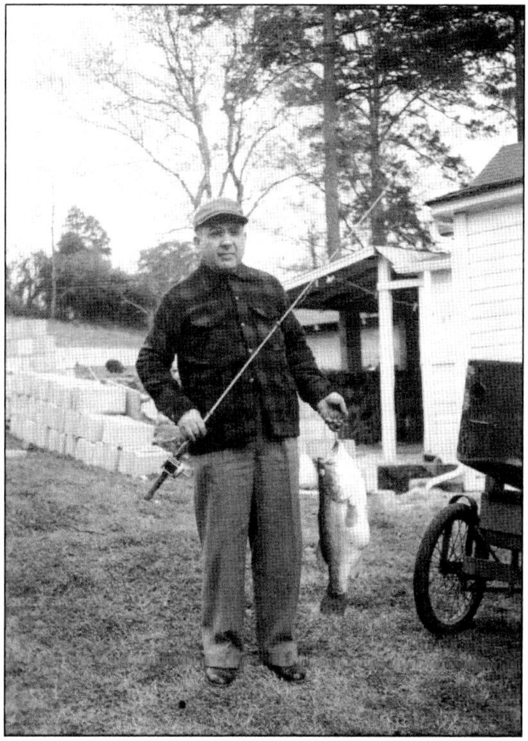

From left to right are Marie Latino, Cheryl Bragg, Donna Bragg, and Rose Bragg. Marie is displaying an eel. Donna and her husband, George Bragg, opened Bragg's Fish Market on Highway 69 in 1962. It is currently operated by their son Mark, who trades in seafood, exotic meats, and cheeses. (Mark Bragg.)

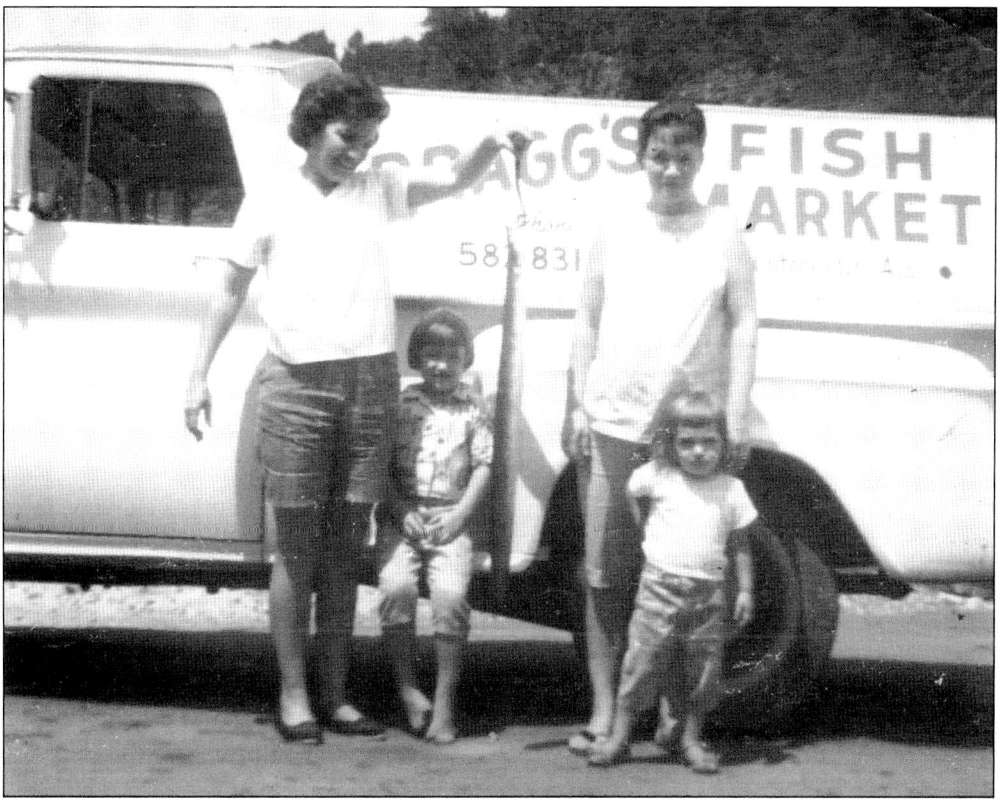

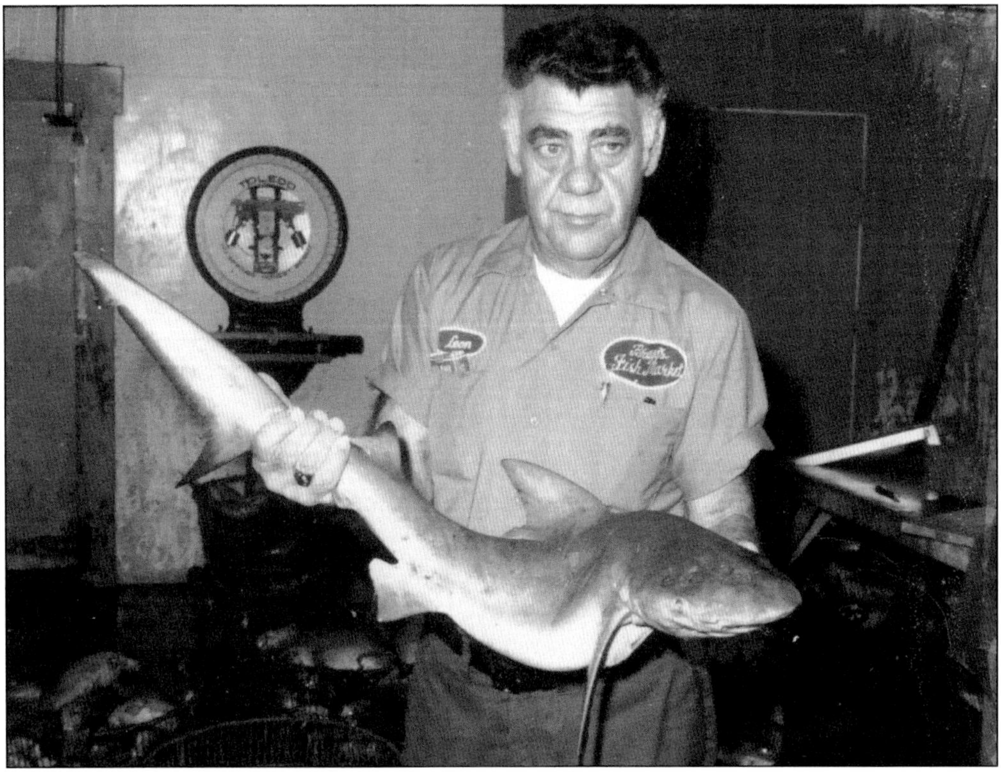

Leon Latino of Bragg's Fish Market is holding a shark. It was not the first or last time a shark or other unusual specimen was discovered in Lake Guntersville. Alligators, sharks, and even piranha have been espied. Since about 14 locks and dams exist between the lake and the gulf, it is certain that rather than swimming here, sharks such as this were released into the lake as a prank. (*Advertiser-Gleam.*)

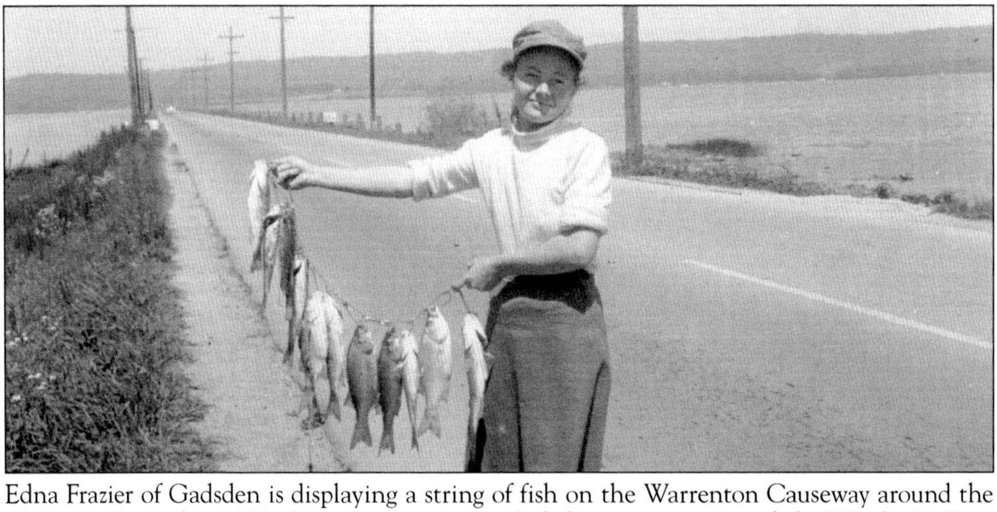

Edna Frazier of Gadsden is displaying a string of fish on the Warrenton Causeway around the 1950s. In December 2016, this causeway was included in a strip renamed the Wright H. Ross Highway. In 1916, Ross made his home in Guntersville, and four years later, he formed the Ross-Graden Lumber Company. Today, this business is run by Wright Ross V, his great-grandson. (Larry Smith.)

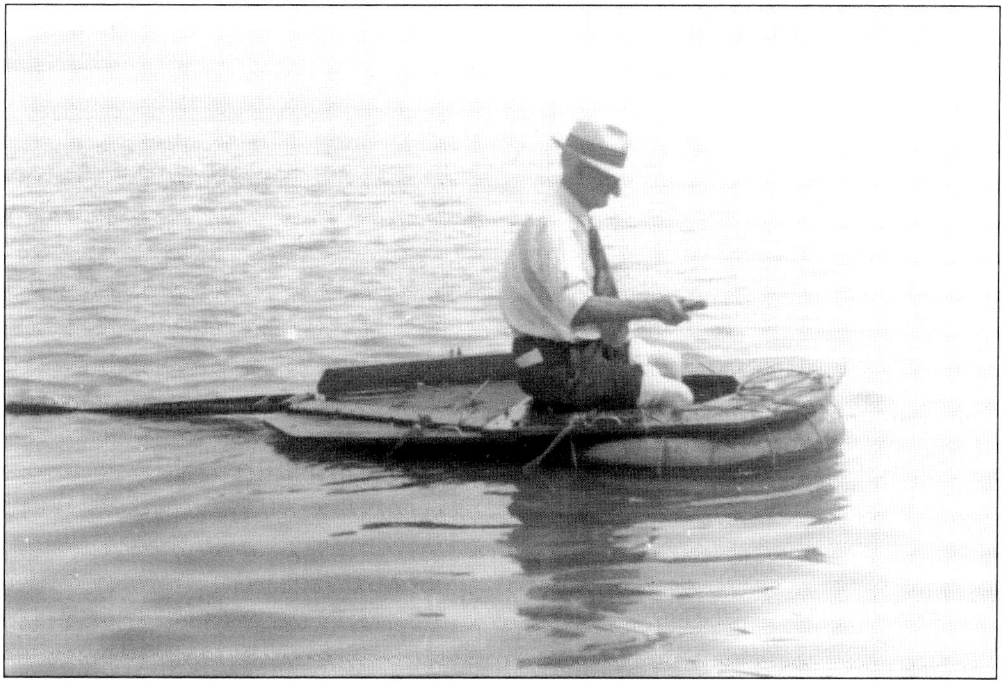

Luther Street Long Sr. is pictured in a duckboat he designed in 1956. Long was an avid sportsman. When he died in 1965, his family donated a "sportsman bookshelf" to the Guntersville Public Library. It was stacked with books on fishing, hunting, and hunting dogs, especially spaniels. (Larry Smith.)

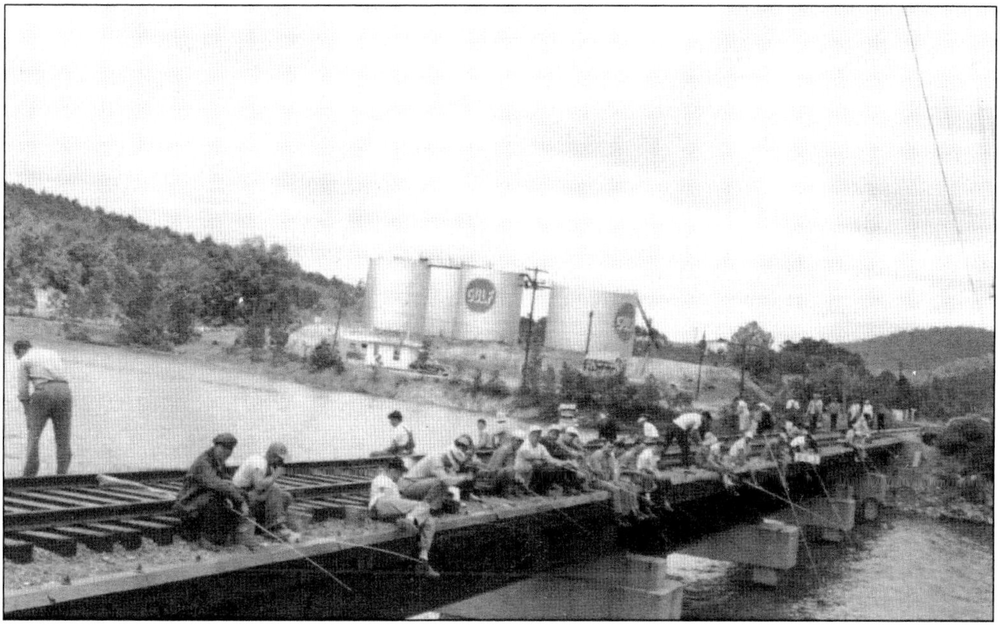

In this c. early-1950s image, people fish on the railroad tracks in Guntersville. Interestingly enough, so often were the tracks congested with fishermen that oncoming trains had to slow down and sometimes stop to avoid collision. Though these individuals are likely locals, by that time, a record number of fishermen flocked to Lake Guntersville. (Larry Smith.)

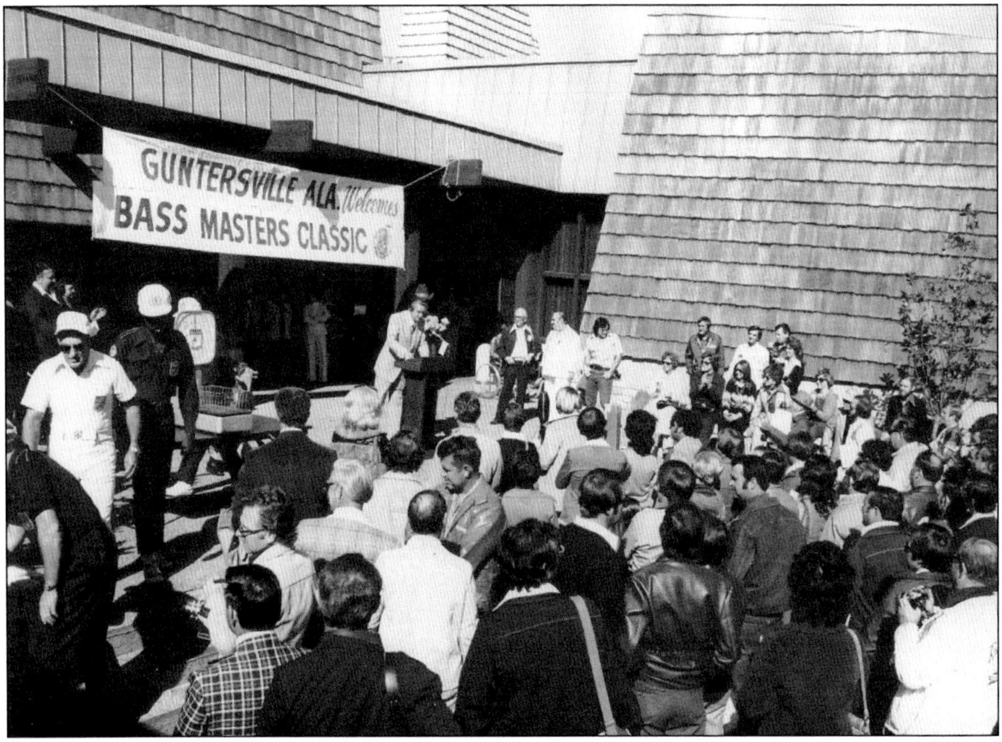

This c. November 1976 image, taken at Guntersville High School, depicts one of many Bassmaster tournaments that have occurred in Guntersville. The champion in 1976 was Rick Clunn, who won $25,000. He said, "This is not a competition between anglers. It's between anglers and the fish." (Top O' The River.)

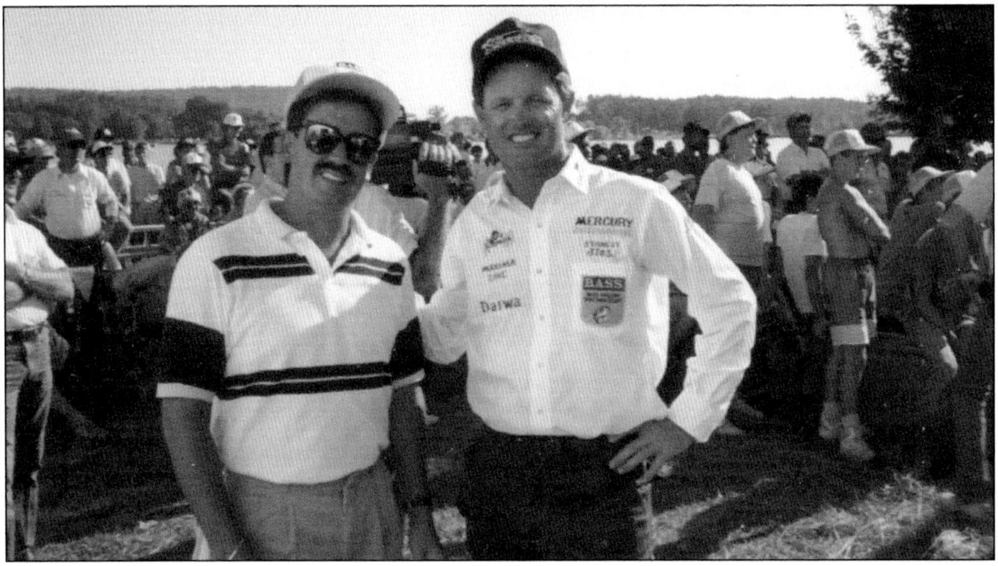

Posing in this photograph are Bubba Martin (left), a director of the Guntersville Chamber of Commerce, and Rick Clunn, winner of the first Bassmaster Classic in Guntersville. The chilly weather and low water levels led Clunn to focus on the creek channels, especially milfoil grass beds. He made his winning catches in Brown's Creek and Beech Creek. (Bubba Martin.)

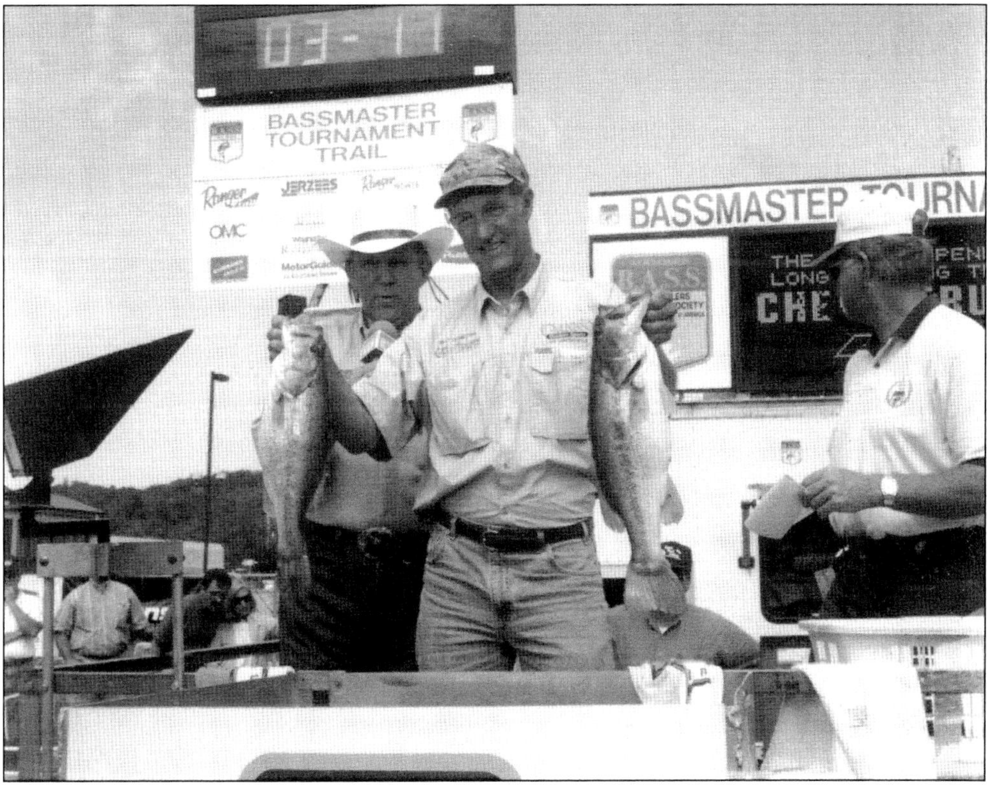

The man holding the fish in this photograph, taken at the 1997 Bassmaster Classic, is Billy Ledbetter of Grant. Ledbetter, a retired Claysville coach who worked at Gann's Outdoors, frequented various fishing tournaments, and he and Phil Gillilan even won an $18,000 bass boat in a Sprint Invitational on Pickwick Lake. (*Advertiser-Gleam*.)

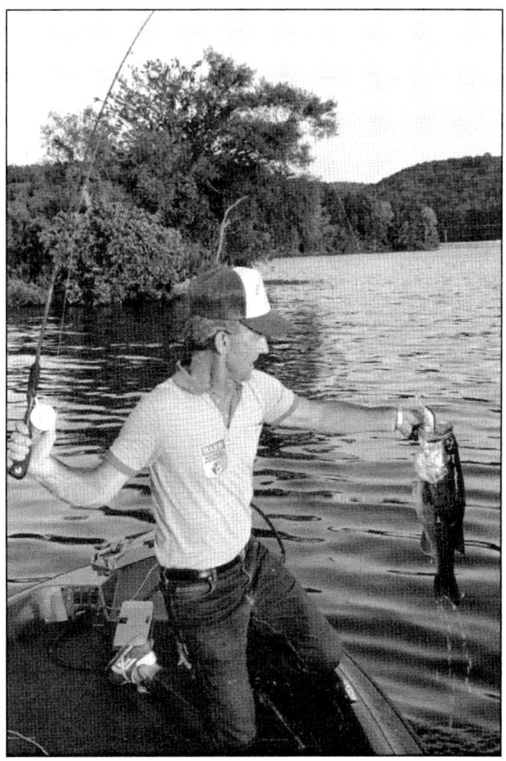

This is Don Snider, an Albertville native, fishing in the Jeff Cook Celebrity Bass Tournament in 1988. Snider and his partner John Horsley of Gadsden won with ten bass that weighed a total of 30.9 pounds. That same year, Snider won first place and $30,000 in the Bass Anglers Sportsman Society's Alabama Invitational in Guntersville. (*Advertiser-Gleam*.)

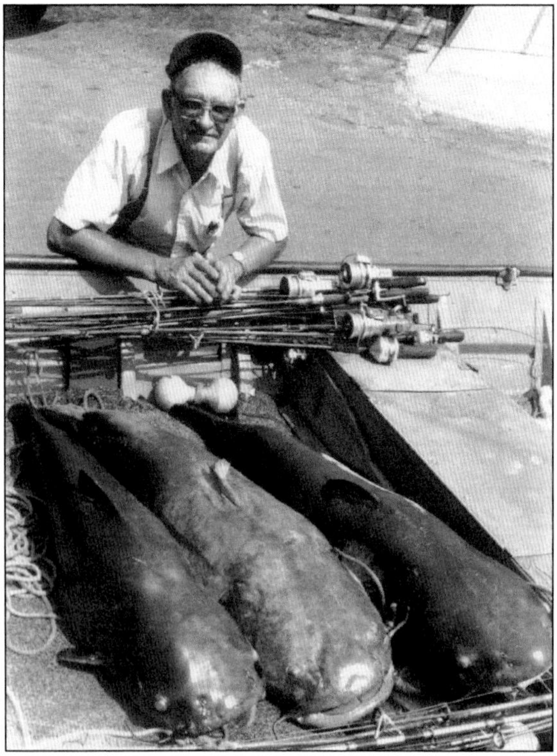

Ralph Lowery, who lived in Albertville, is pictured with three large catfish that weighed 53, 75, and 65 pounds. He caught all three in about half an hour while fishing on Lake Guntersville. Unfortunately, he lacked a dip net, but a nearby fisherman saw his dilemma and loaned him one. (*Advertiser-Gleam.*)

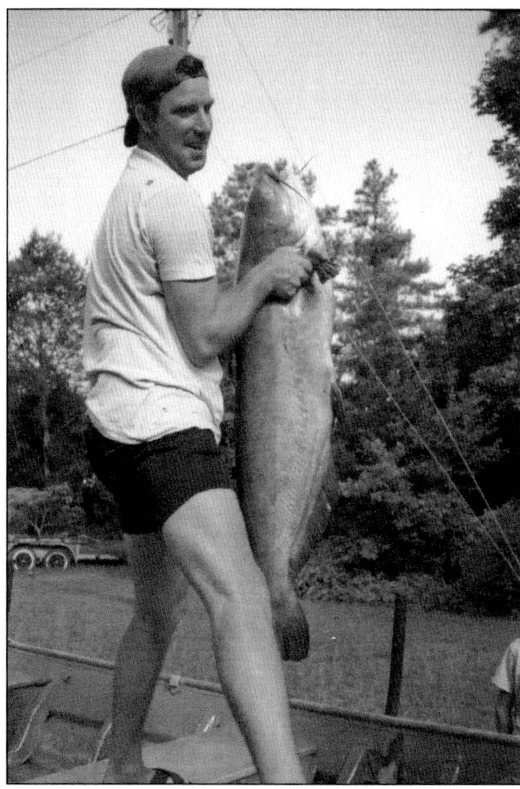

Dale Hill (shown here), a resident of Snow Point Road, spent over 30 years as a commercial fisherman in Guntersville. Unsurprisingly, he has caught myriad lunkers. In 1994, he caught this 96-pound catfish on a rod and reel below the Tennessee Valley Authority Guntersville Dam. He and his wife, Kathy, have two children, Frances and James. (Authors' collection.)

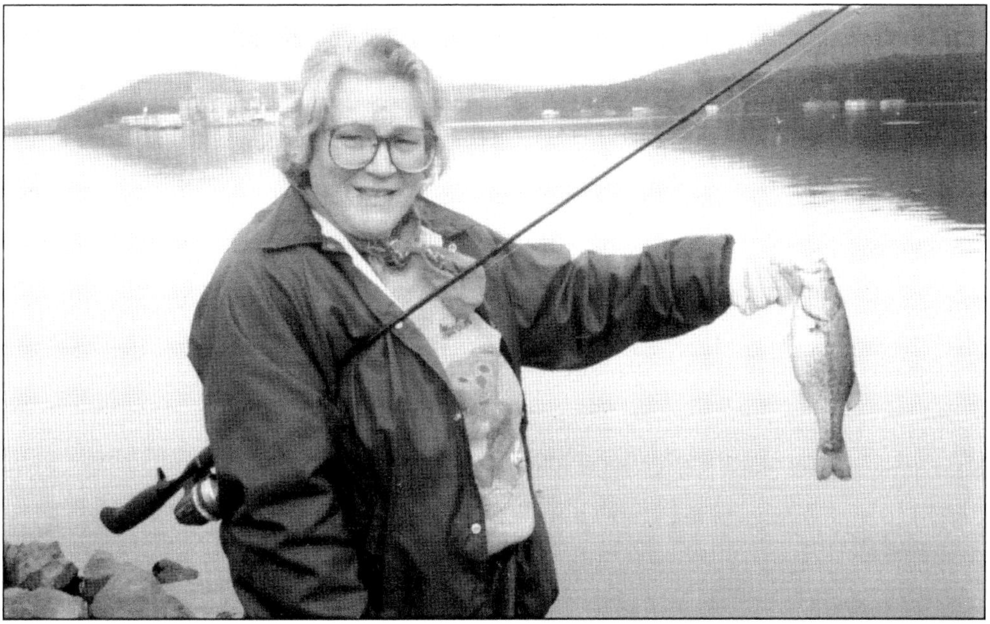

Susie Hutchinson of Guntersville is holding a small bass while fishing on Lake Guntersville around 1993. One of her best catches took place in 1989 when, while fishing with her grandson C.R. Dotson, she caught three bass weighing 4.75, 6, and 8.9 pounds. The feed mill can be seen in the background. (*Advertiser-Gleam.*)

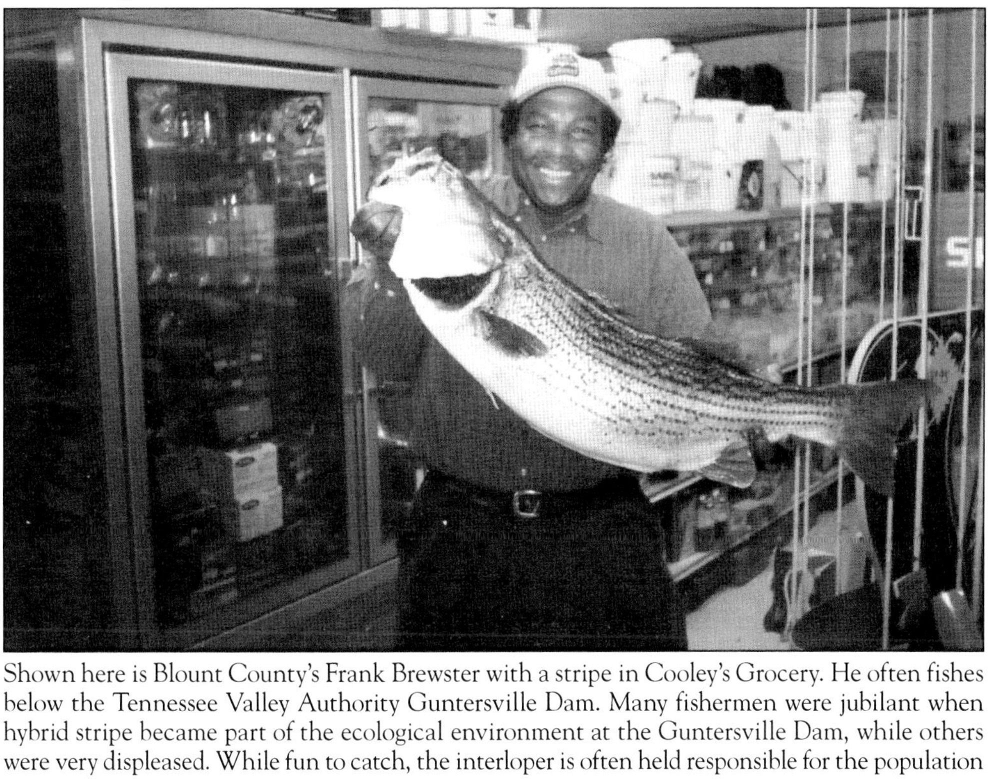

Shown here is Blount County's Frank Brewster with a stripe in Cooley's Grocery. He often fishes below the Tennessee Valley Authority Guntersville Dam. Many fishermen were jubilant when hybrid stripe became part of the ecological environment at the Guntersville Dam, while others were very displeased. While fun to catch, the interloper is often held responsible for the population decrease of sauger. (Tony Cooley.)

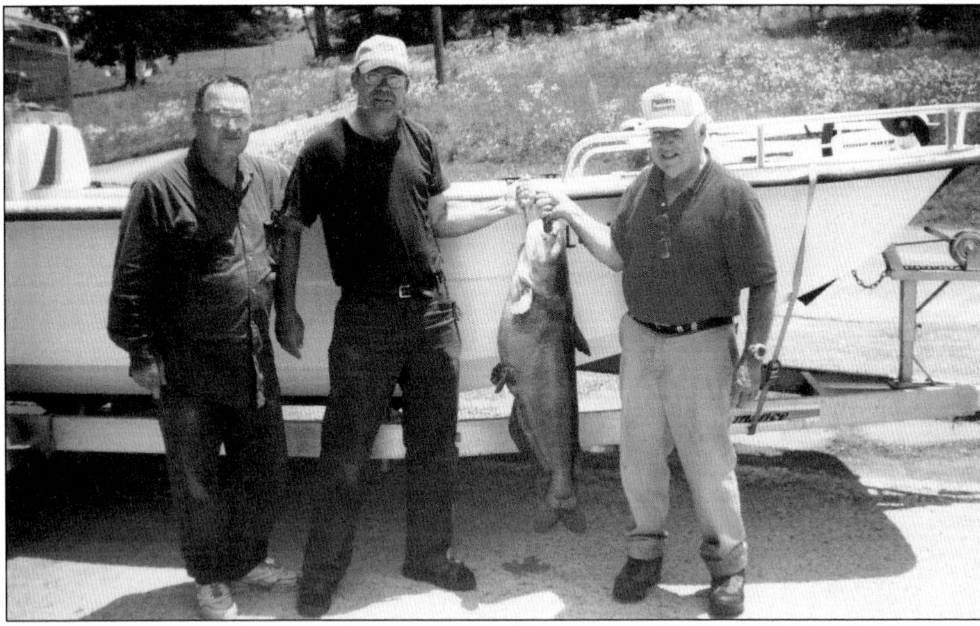

From left to right are Glen McNeil, Ron Hyatt, and Dr. Hampton E. "Sonny" Barker. Barker served in the US Army and the Alabama National Guard. A graduate of the University of Alabama, he opened a dental practice in Arab in 1965. He and his wife, Nancy, had a son, Andrew "Bucky," and two daughters, Catharine and Aimee. Dr. Barker died in 2015. (Tony Cooley.)

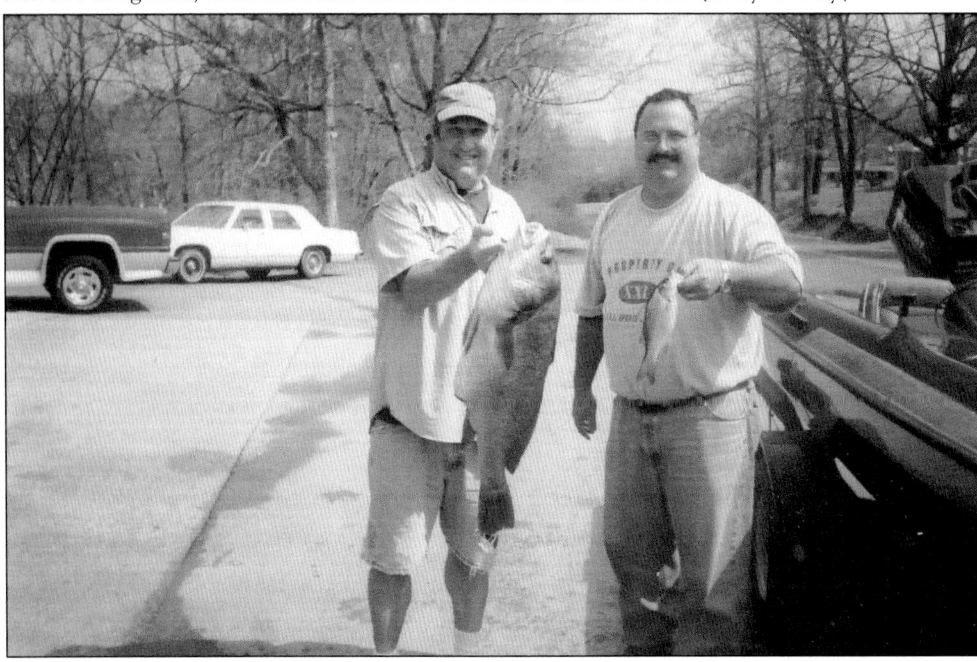

John Townsend (left) of Union Grove and Ronny Shumate of Arab are comparing catches outside of Tony Cooley's Grocery. Townsend's daughter Jackie married Shumate's son Clint. The two are proud grandfathers to Harper Rose Shumate. Townsend and his wife, Jeannette, have three other daughters: Kelly, Kerry, and Joni. Ronny and his wife, Denice, also have a son named Cody. (Tony Cooley).

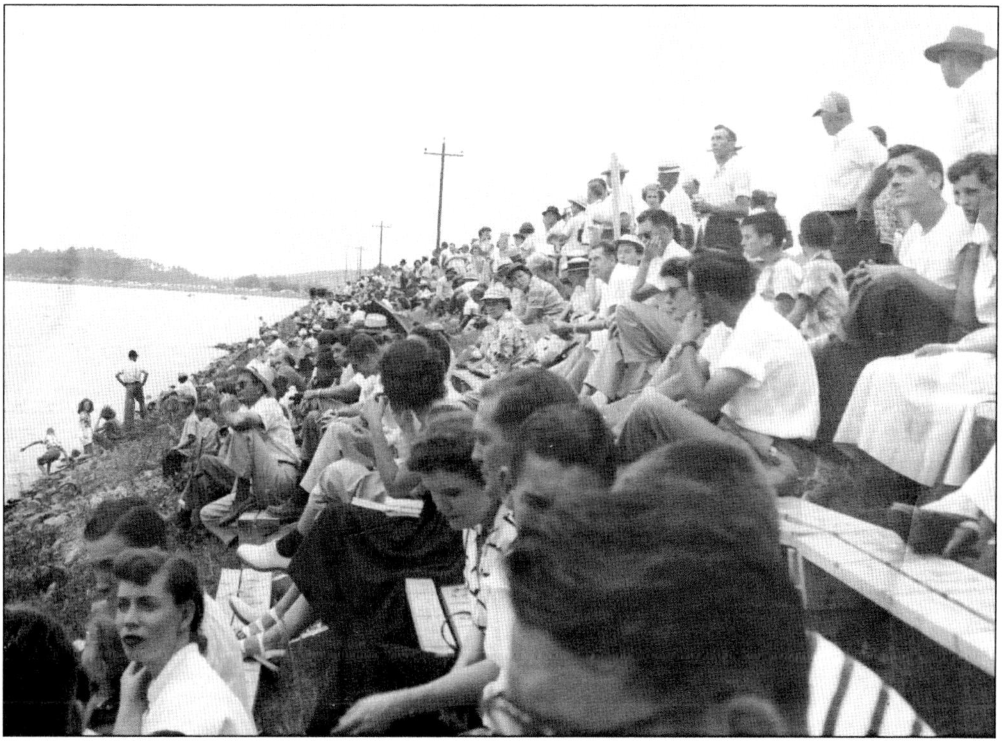

The boat race project required a monumental number of volunteer hours. The annual event needed financial and logistical organization and planning. Over the years, the whole town was abuzz with excitement about gaining national fame. Many locals attended out of curiosity, while others sought entertainment. The races did not disappoint. (Guntersville Museum.)

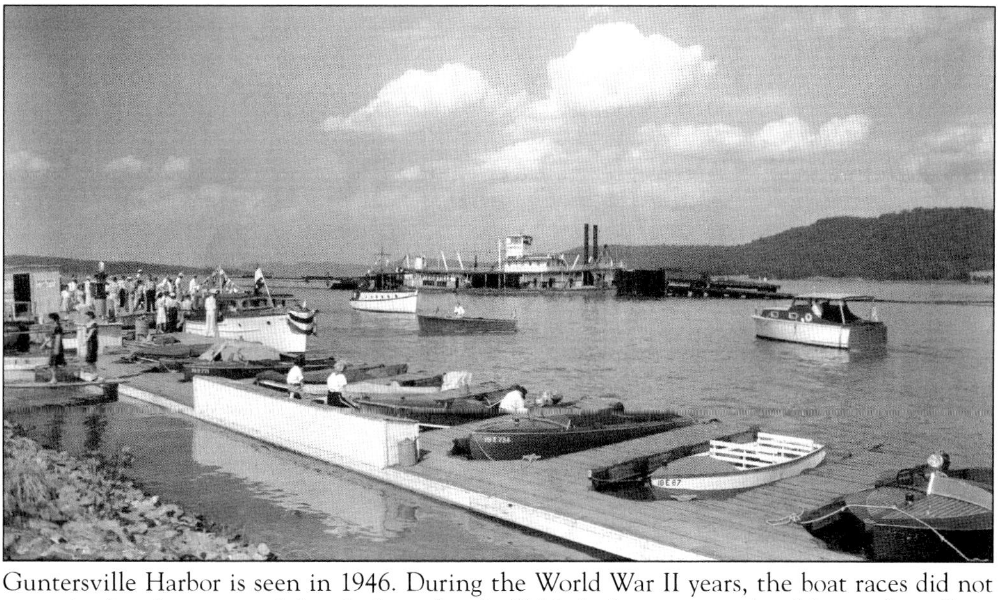

Guntersville Harbor is seen in 1946. During the World War II years, the boat races did not transpire, but they resumed shortly thereafter. In 1946, the boat race weekend featured a sailboat race and the Borden Jones ski troupe. There were so many boat race contestants that year that the local newspaper beseeched locals to offer rooms in their homes. (David Jones.)

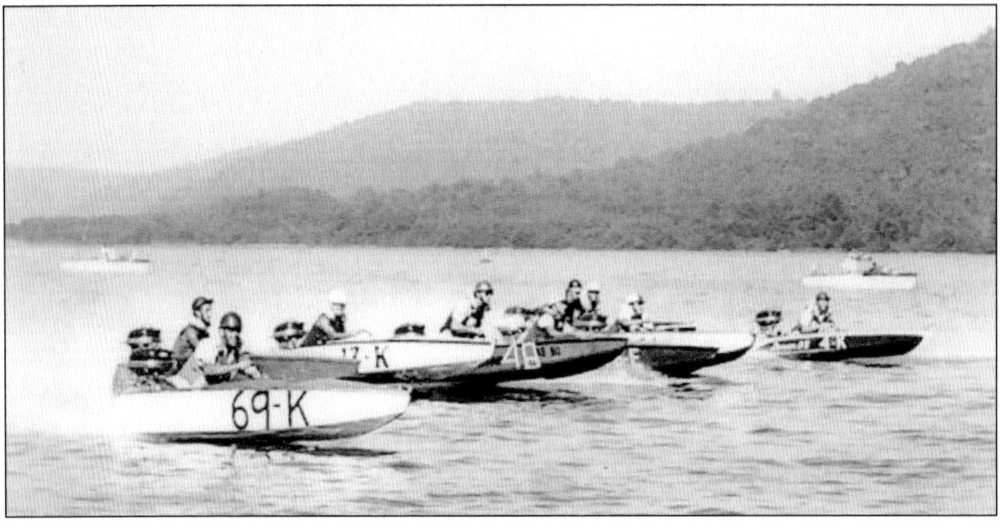

This c. 1951 image is from one of the early boat races on Lake Guntersville. Over the years, the location and length of the racecourse changed. Different divisions and categories were also added. Local, state, and national press coverage skyrocketed, and each year seemed to have more tourists than the last. (Guntersville Museum.)

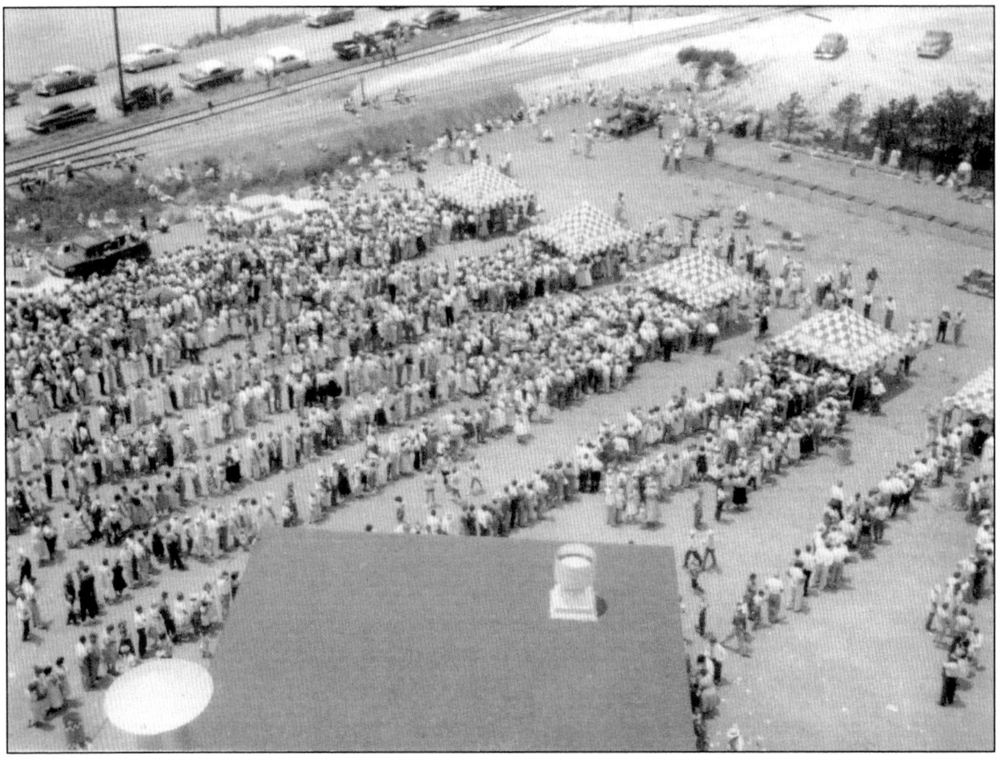

As shown in this c. 1950s photograph, crowds descended on Lake Guntersville during the boat races. Local businesses, especially hotels, motels, and restaurants, benefited from a rush of customers. Though the boat races provided entertainment and brought tourist dollars to the area, some locals nevertheless disliked the traffic and chose not to go out on boat race weekends. (Gail Smith Ingrum.)

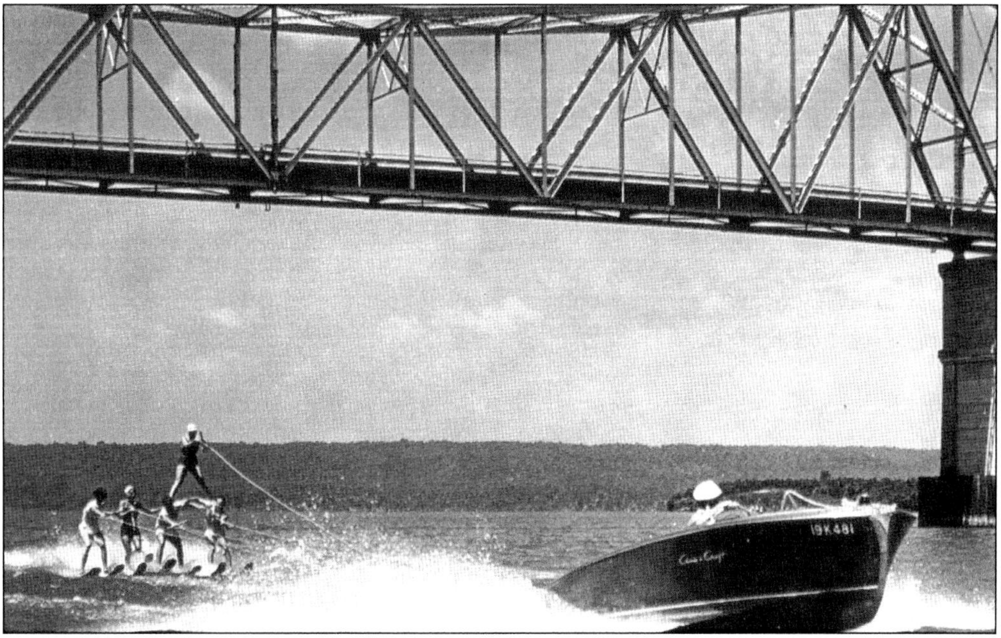

Often accompanying the boat races were water performances, especially those showcasing skiing. Various stunts delighted crowd members, many of whom cheered while gazing in wonderment. In addition to aquatic entertainment, the boat races included a contest for the best decorated boat. The 1948 winner was Clay Woodall. (George Barnett.)

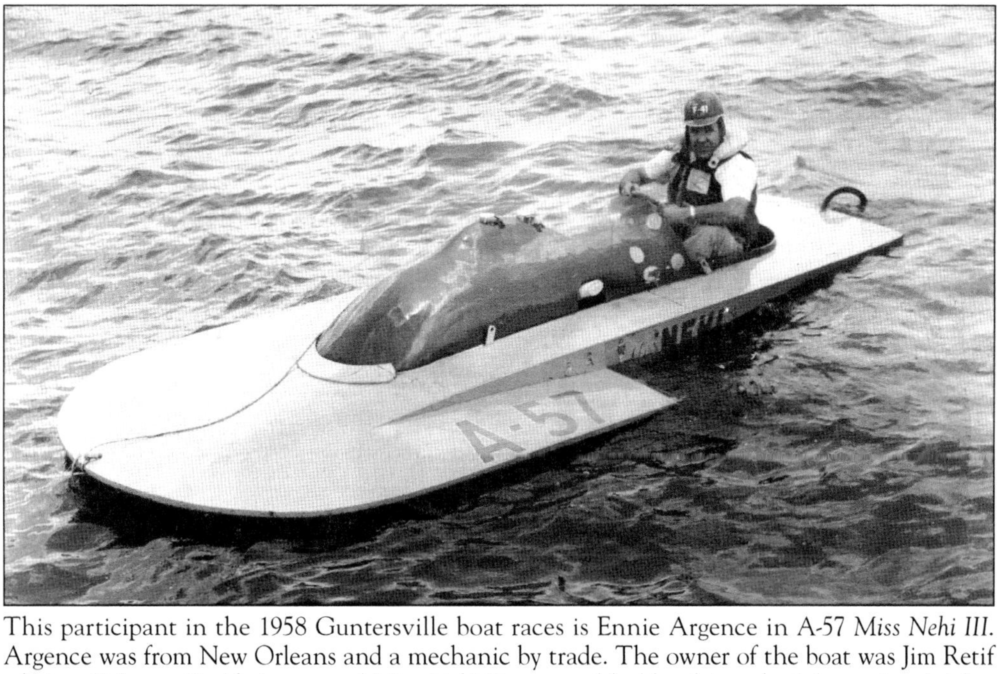

This participant in the 1958 Guntersville boat races is Ennie Argence in A-57 *Miss Nehi III*. Argence was from New Orleans and a mechanic by trade. The owner of the boat was Jim Retif of New Orleans. Retif also owned *Miss Nehi II*, a record holder driven by Johnny Landaiche. (Marshall County Archives.)

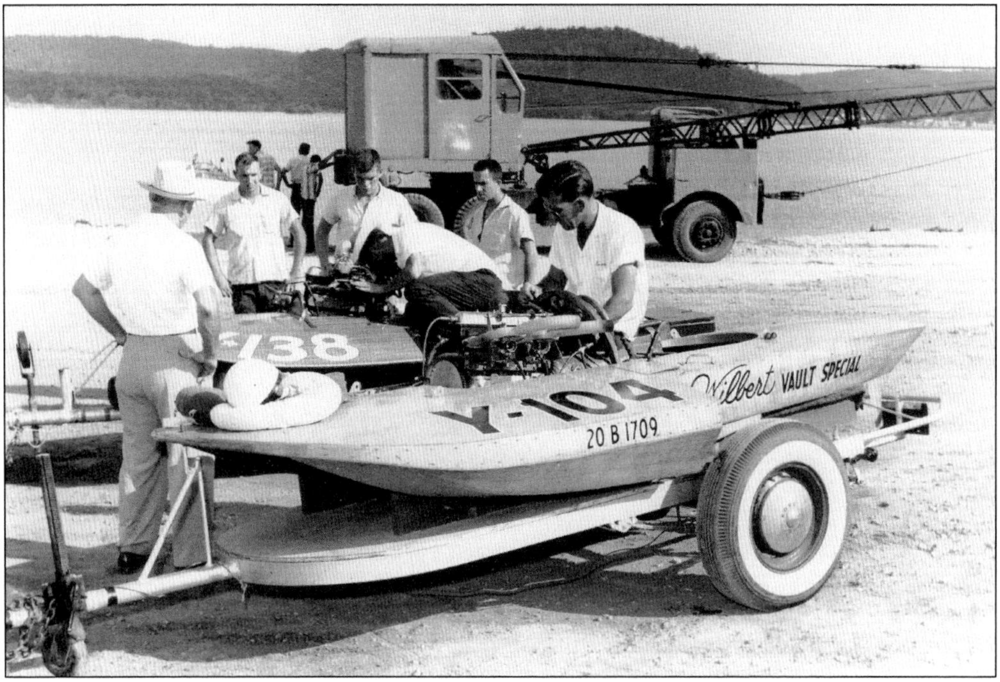

In 1960, Milton Gagnon, a driver from New Orleans, won the first heat of the 266-cubic-inch hydroplane race in *My Security*. In the second event, Gagnon flipped his boat and was trapped. Quick efforts by the crash patrol prevented his drowning. Top honors went to Ennie Argence (front right), shown working on a boat. (Guntersville Historical Society.)

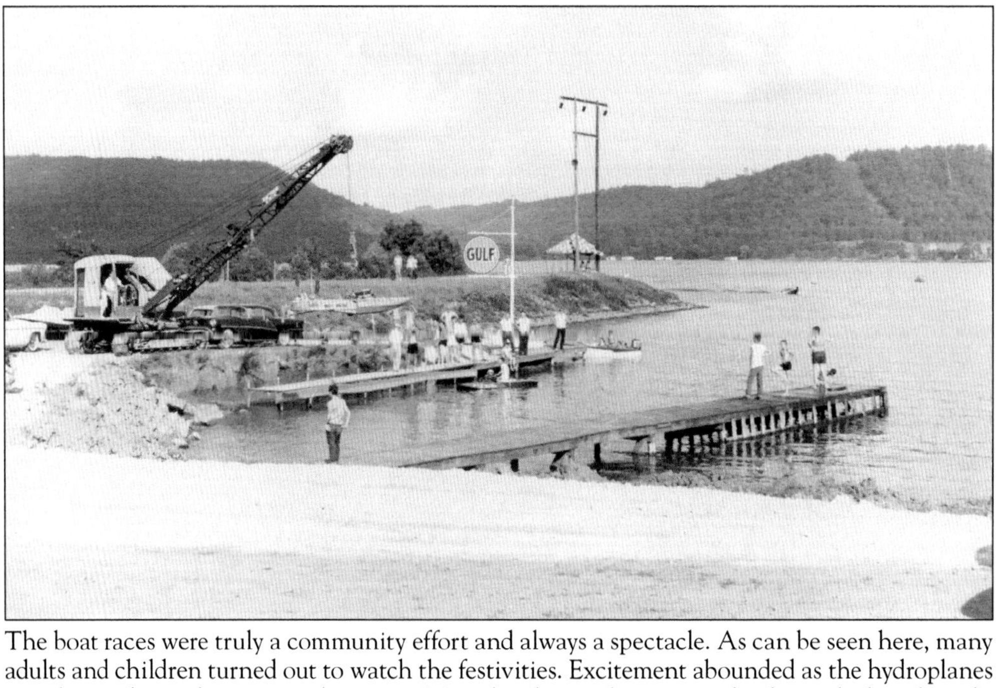

The boat races were truly a community effort and always a spectacle. As can be seen here, many adults and children turned out to watch the festivities. Excitement abounded as the hydroplanes were lowered into the water with a crane. Many locals eagerly attempted to learn the boat brands, models, sponsors, and drivers. (Marshall County Archives.)

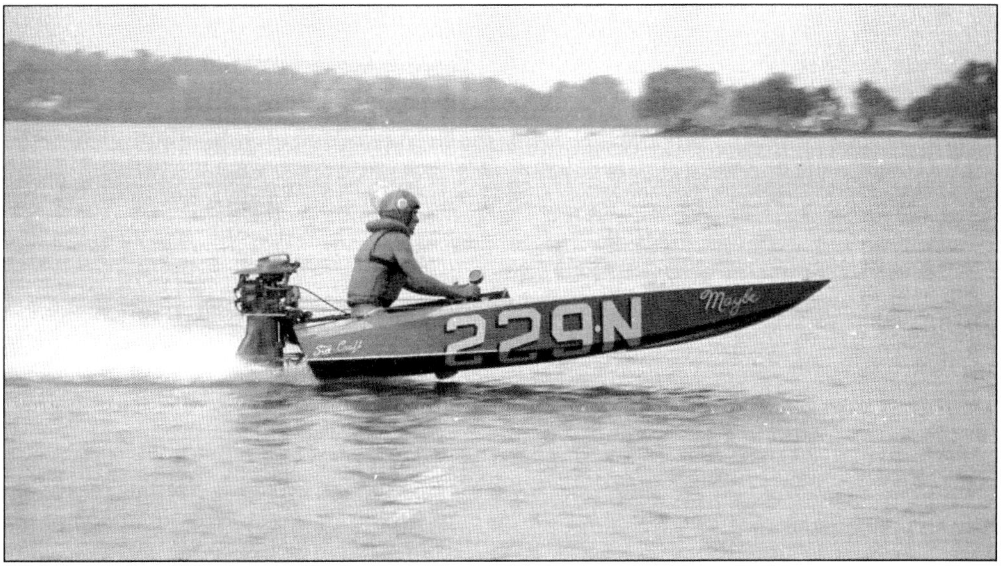

This is an unidentified participant in an undated photograph of the Guntersville boat races. The name of the boat is *Maybe*. In 1960, the Guntersville Jaycees actually thought about ending the event. Cost was the main concern. In 1959, the races made $10,000, but after expenses, the Jaycees were left with only a $1,000 profit. (Marshall County Archives.)

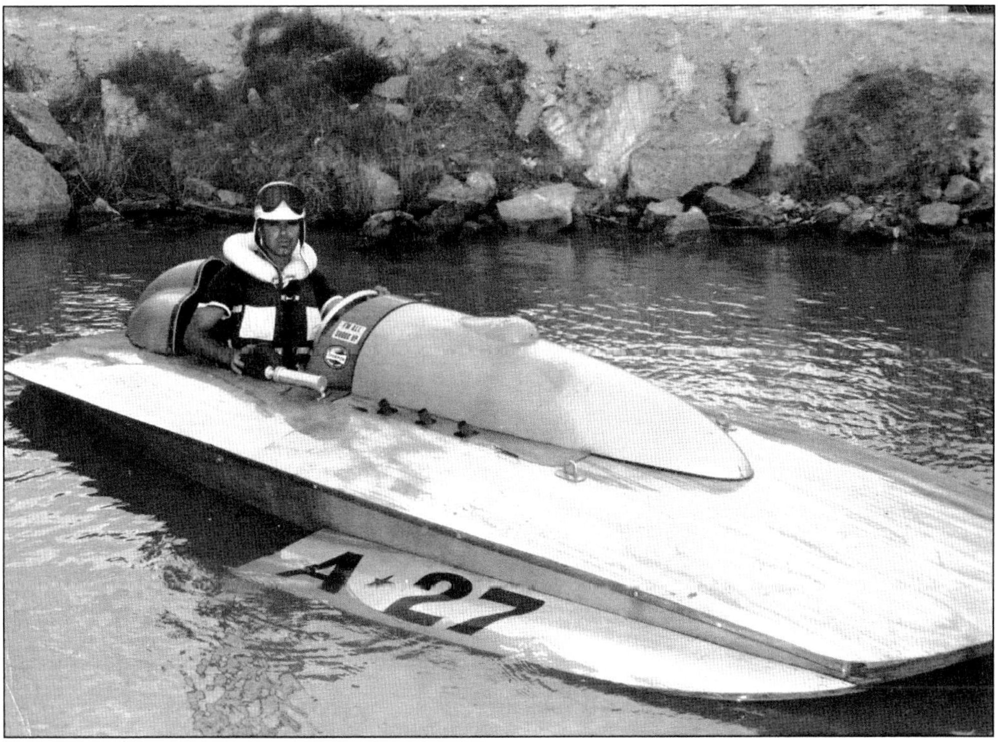

Another unidentified participant is pictured in an undated photograph from the Guntersville boat races. A sticker on his boat reads, "I'm all shook up." The Jaycees' financial concerns were founded, for in 1961, the boat races lost money, specifically $2,073. This was blamed on the expense of trophies and monetary prizes. (Marshall County Archives.)

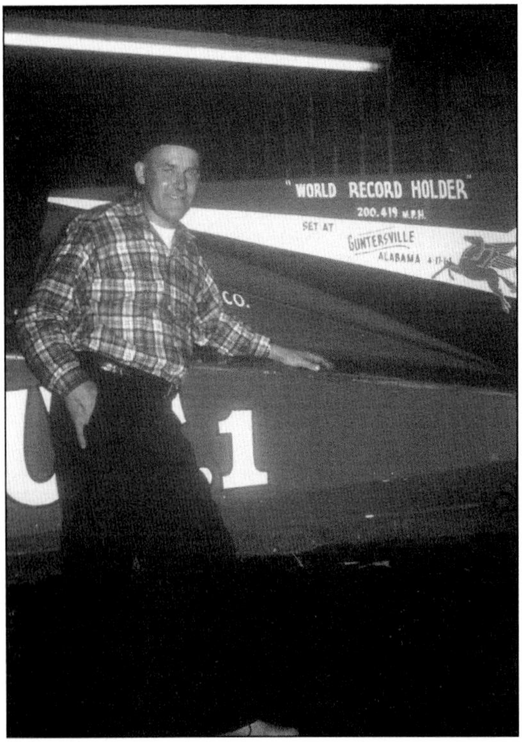
"WORLD RECORD HOLDER"
200.419 M.P.H.
SET AT
GUNTERSVILLE
ALABAMA

Roy Duby, a native of Detroit, Michigan, set a world speedboat record of 200.419 miles per hour while driving *Miss U.S. I* on Lake Guntersville on April 17, 1962. The Jaycees were thrilled that this accomplishment attracted attention to Guntersville. The previous record holder was Bill Muncey of Seattle, Washington. Muncey had achieved 192.001 miles per hour. (Guntersville Historical Society.)

Six members of the Guntersville Jaycees help racer Roy Duby polish his award-winning boat *Miss U.S. I*. From left to right are (seated) Reese Burns and Jackie Doyle Harris; (standing) Hugh Burgess Jr., Dickie Cheatham, Jerry Nabors, and Buddy Taylor. (Larry Smith.)

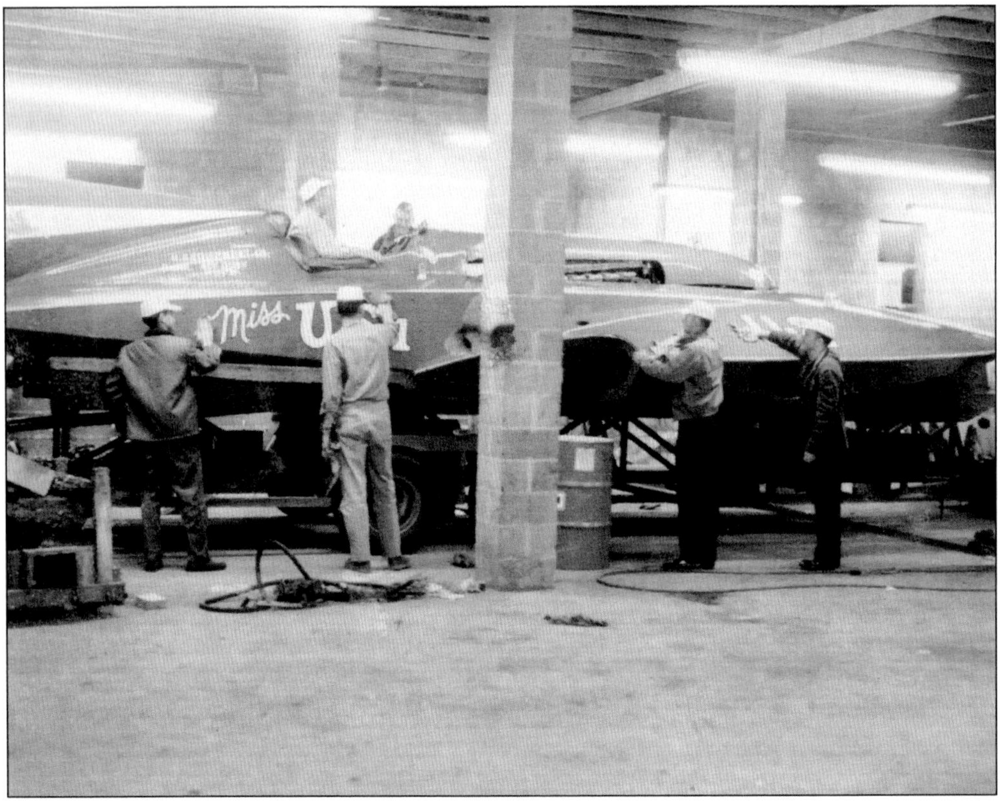

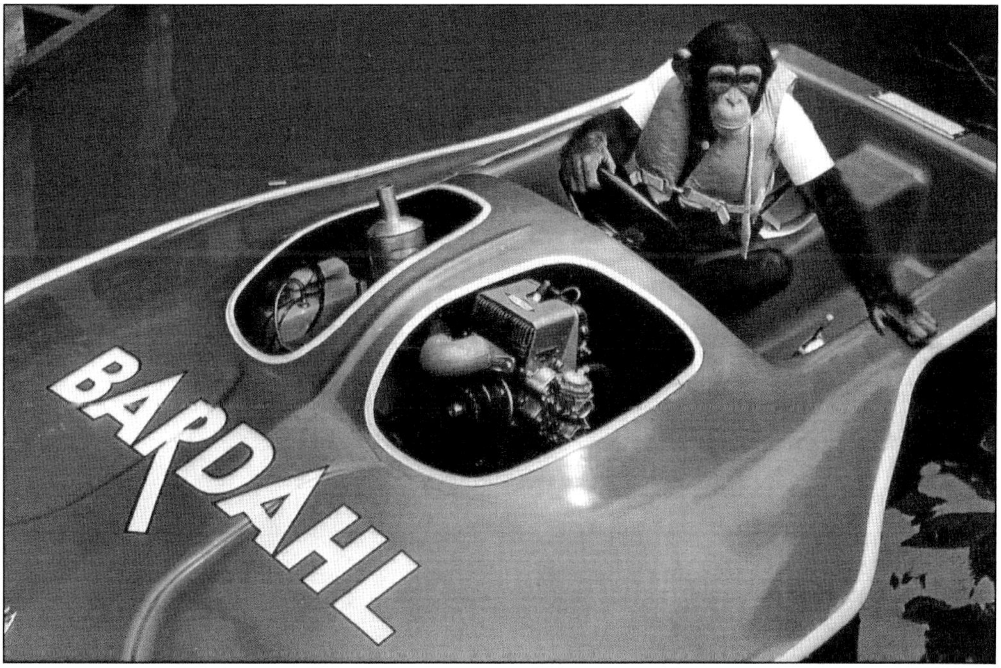

Poncho, a chimpanzee belonging to Guntersville's Rip Barnett, is shown sitting in a tiny boat as publicity for the boat races in 1963. This photograph was sent to various newspapers and magazines, although the boat race committee mulled over possible captions. Cochair Mort Epstein mused, "Guntersville has gone ape over the boat races." (George Barnett.)

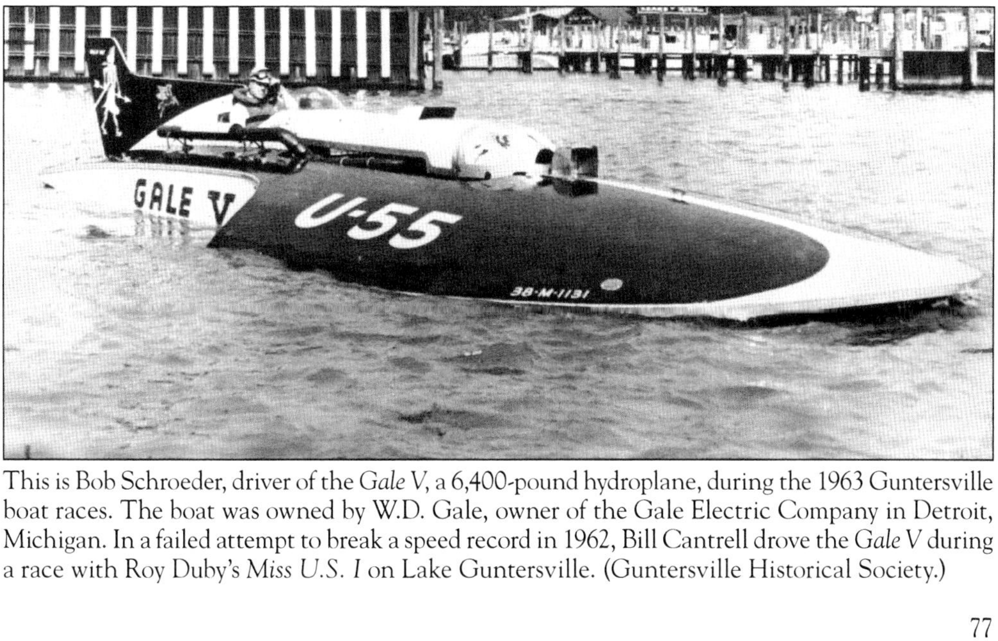

This is Bob Schroeder, driver of the *Gale V*, a 6,400-pound hydroplane, during the 1963 Guntersville boat races. The boat was owned by W.D. Gale, owner of the Gale Electric Company in Detroit, Michigan. In a failed attempt to break a speed record in 1962, Bill Cantrell drove the *Gale V* during a race with Roy Duby's *Miss U.S. I* on Lake Guntersville. (Guntersville Historical Society.)

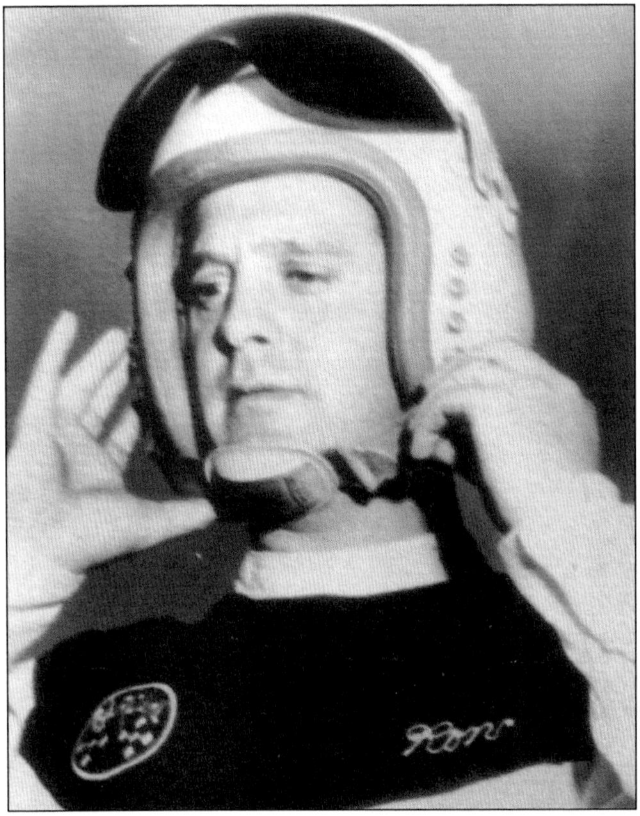

Ron Musson was a winner in the 1963 Alabama Governor's Cup at Guntersville. Between 1959 and 1963, he won 16 out of 47 boat races. He was well known for driving the hydroplanes *Hawaii Kai III*, *Nitrogen Too*, and *Miss Bardahl*. Sadly, Musson died in 1966 when his boat crashed during a race. (Marshall County Archives.)

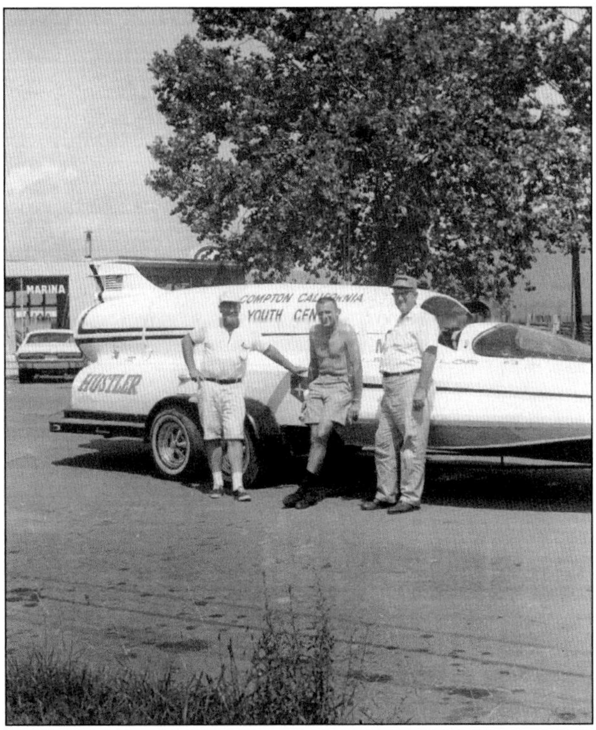

From left to right are Pete Duncan (marina owner), Hoot Word, and Paul Holland. They are standing in front of *The Hustler*, which, driven by Lee Taylor, won the water speedboat record on Lake Guntersville in June 1967. The previous record was 277.33 miles per hour, and Taylor achieved 285.21 miles per hour. (Marshall County Archives.)

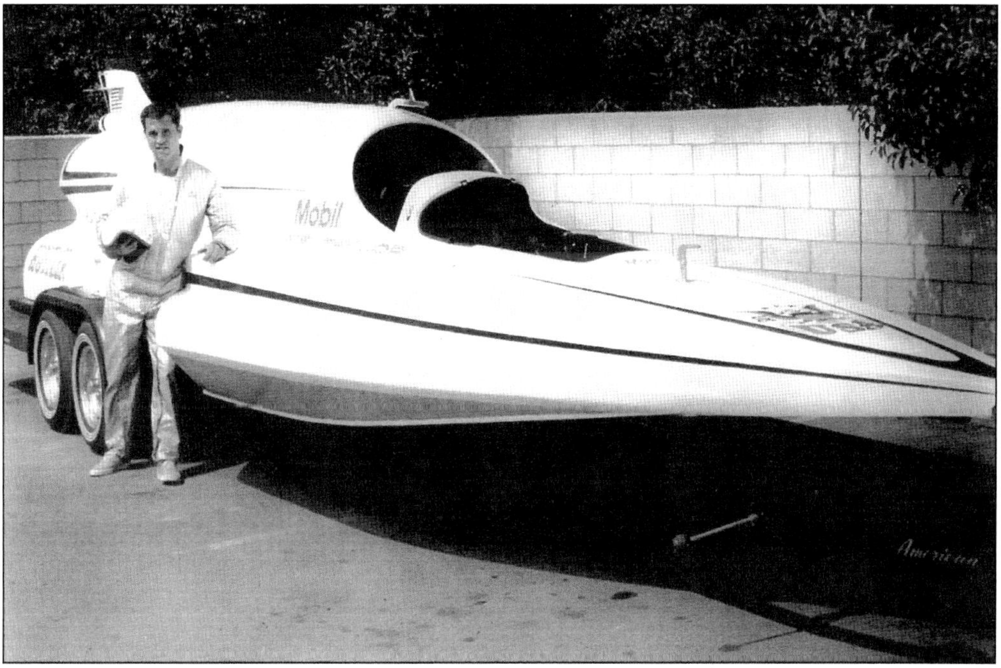

Lee Taylor poses with *The Hustler*. He was from Downey, California, and a hobbyist boat racer. He had tried to break the speed record in 1966 but only achieved 230.317 miles per hour. When he broke the speed record in 1967, his boat was displayed for days at Park Avenue and Forty-Eighth Street in New York City. (Guntersville Historical Society.)

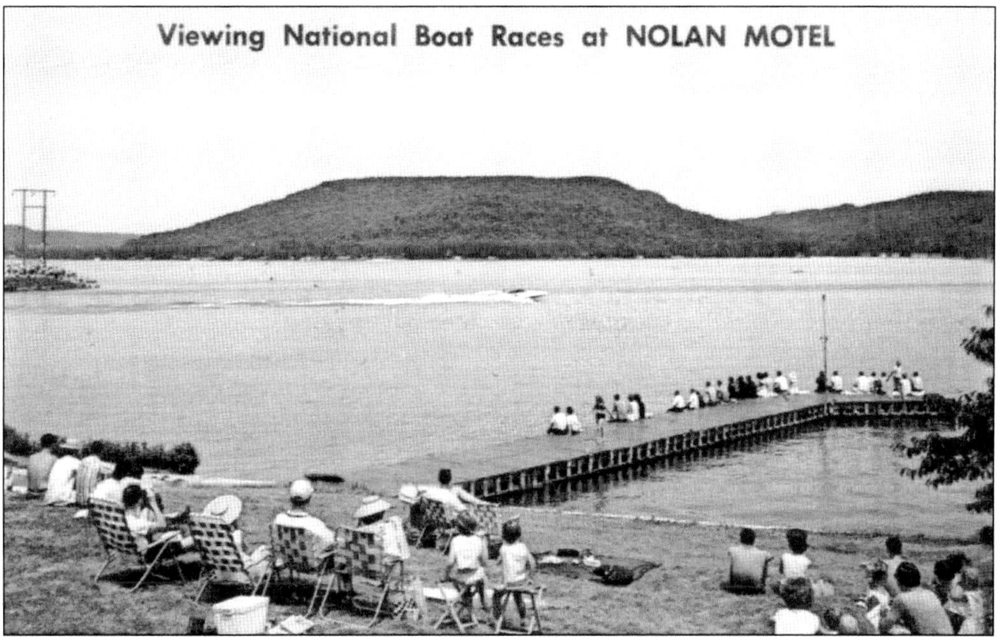

This postcard shows spectators enjoying the Guntersville boat races from the Nolan Motel. Opened in 1960, the motel was advertised as having 22 rooms, a restaurant with an experienced chef, and conference facilities. The motel lasted until March 1984, when it was leveled to make room for a Holiday Inn. (Marshall County Archives.)

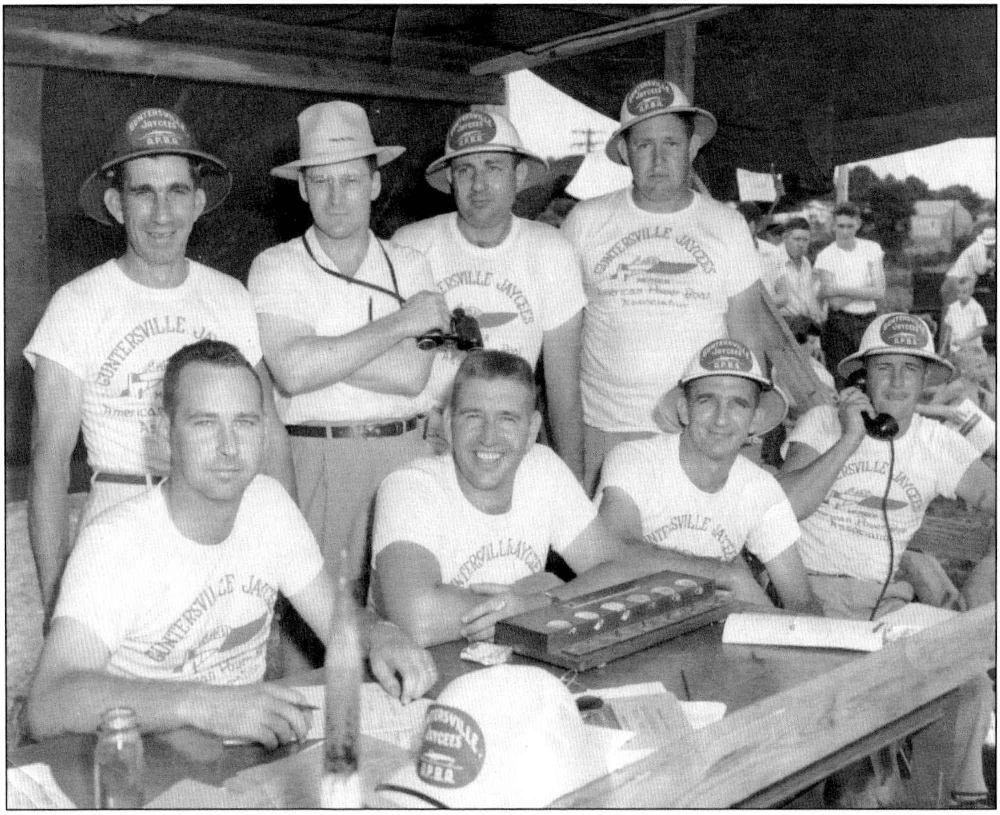

These Guntersville Jaycee members are watching an undated boat race on Lake Guntersville. From left to right are (seated) Ray Dunlap, Charlie Pass, Walter Posey, and Claude Herbert Smith; (standing) Buel Locklear, Dr. Lowell Bechart, Ray Ogletree, and Clayton Carter. (Gail Smith Ingrum.)

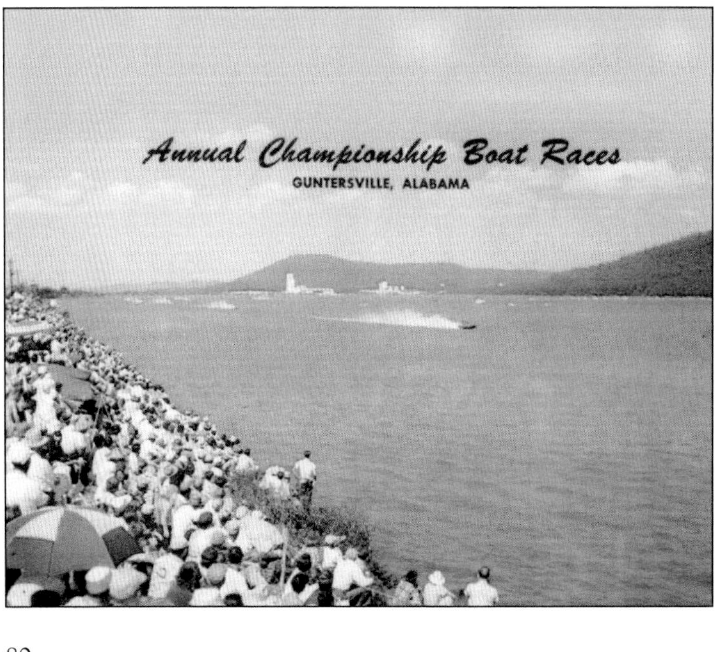

Because the Dixie Cup boat races contributed greatly to Guntersville's tourism economy, a variety of postcards like this one were sold to locals and visitors alike. Some show the hydroplanes, while others depict the enthusiastic crowds watching the races or enjoying the festivities and concessions. (Guntersville Museum.)

This sign used to sit north of the George Houston Bridge in Guntersville. From left to right are Ulwyne Harrell Hefferman, Joe Segler, and Jo Starnes. Guntersville locals embraced the nickname "Playground of the South," and it was used in pamphlets, advertisements, and radio broadcasts. At one point, a motel called Playground of the South was located on US Highway 431. (Jo Starnes Goss.)

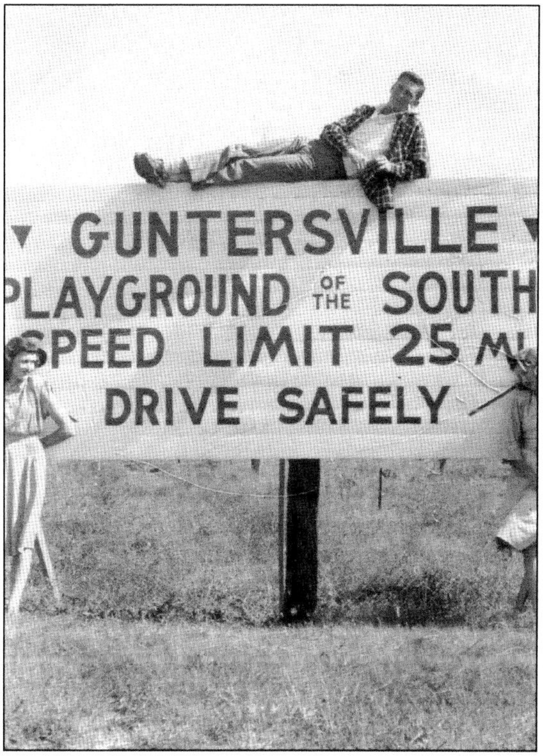
GUNTERSVILLE
PLAYGROUND OF THE SOUTH
SPEED LIMIT 25
DRIVE SAFELY

Pleasure boats have always been a familiar sight on Lake Guntersville. Then as now, it is a popular location for sightseers, who often travel from far and wide. Whether taking a speedy or leisurely pace over the waters, locals and tourists basked in the lake's beauty. (Marshall County Archives.)

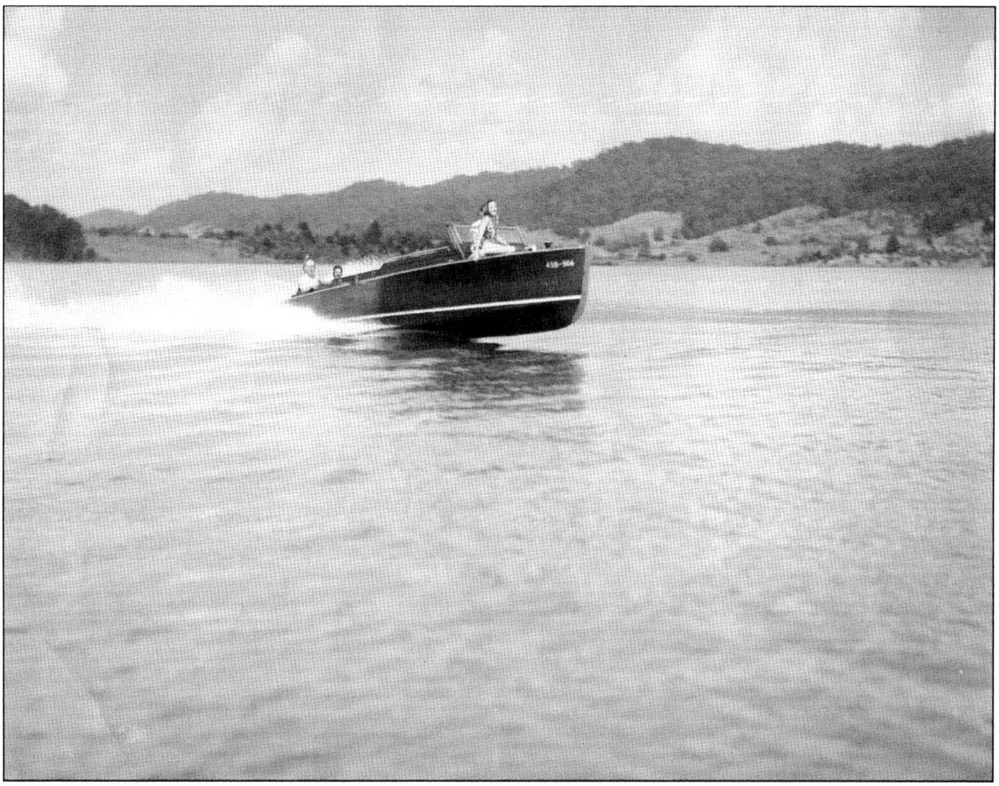

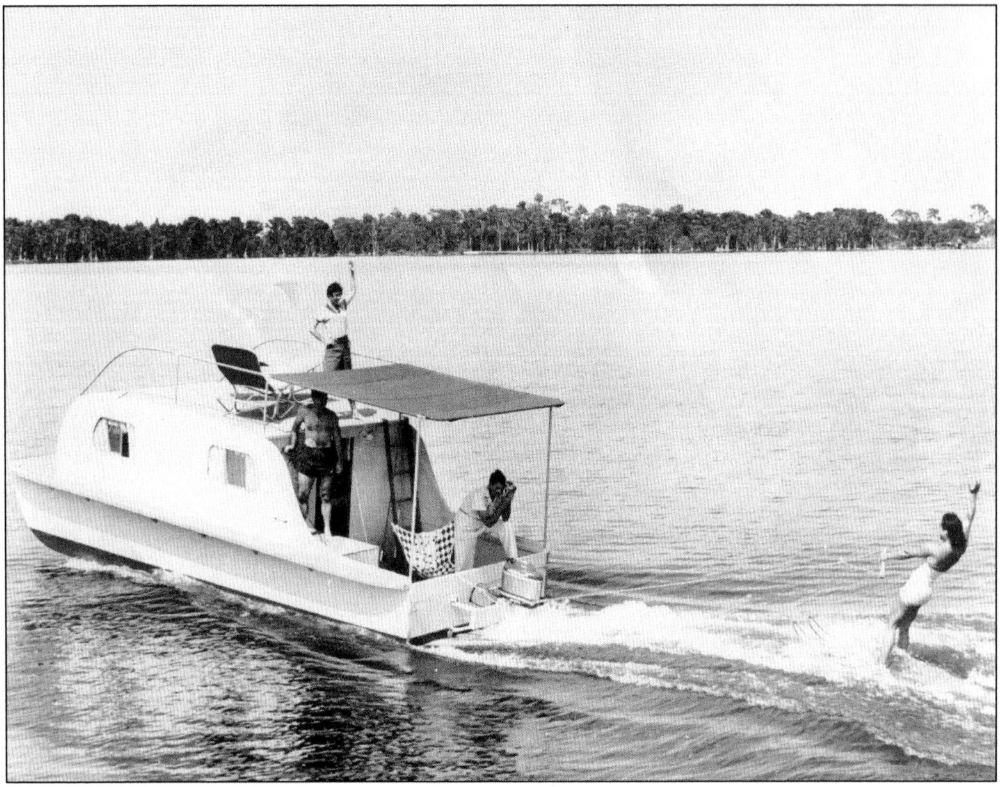

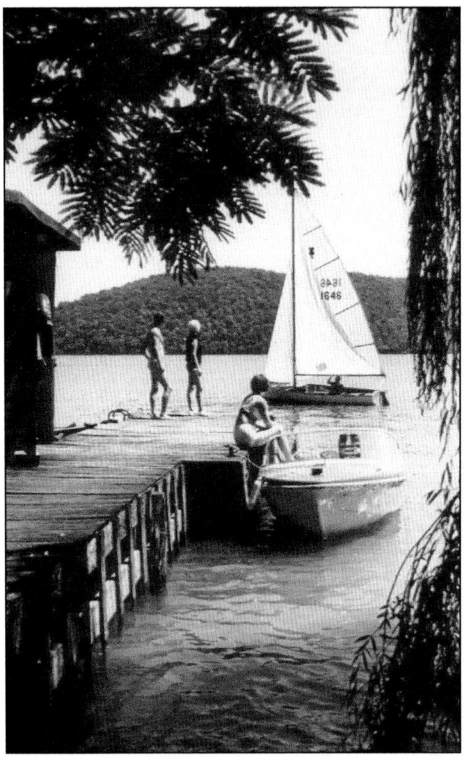

Skiing is a favorite pastime on Lake Guntersville. At one time, exhibitions of skiing talent including kite flying, jumping, slalom, barefoot skiing, and even "death-defying" tricks were offered as water spectaculars. Individuals and ski clubs participated in competitions sponsored by civic groups as fundraisers. (Larry Smith.)

Throughout the summer, sailboats abound on Lake Guntersville. In 1959, the Lake Guntersville Yacht Club began sponsoring an annual Harvest Regatta, which attracted sailboats not only from Alabama but also from nearby states like Georgia, Tennessee, Mississippi, and Louisiana, as well as from distant states like California. (Marshall County Archives.)

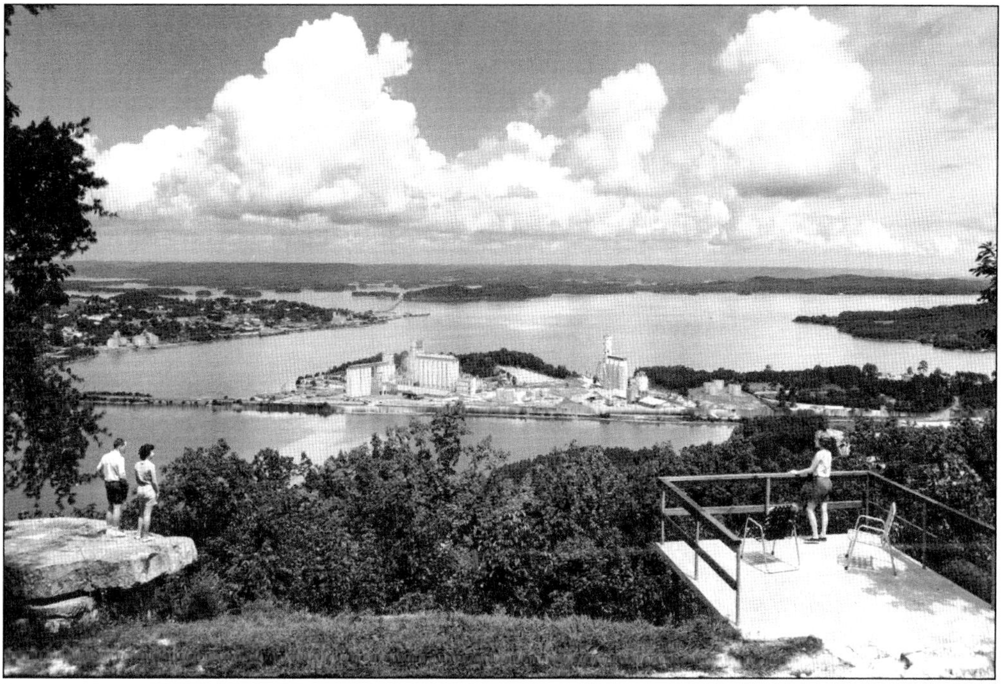

These teenagers are viewing Lake Guntersville from Wyeth Rock. From left to right are Randy Laney, Judy Starnes, and Milla McCord. Today, the large building in the middle is the Wayne Farms Feed Mill. Bream fishing is spectacular near the mill. It is located on Lake Guntersville Drive on the route to Lake Guntersville State Park. (*Advertiser-Gleam*.)

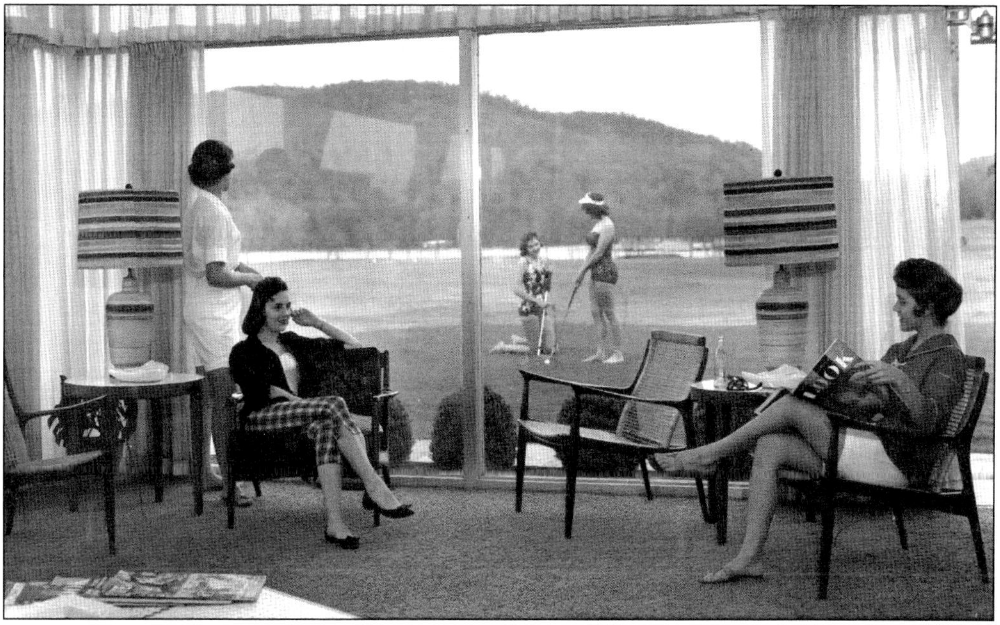

These unidentified women are relaxing at the Val Monte Shores resort in Guntersville. It opened on May 4, 1958, and had a pool, two golf courses, a clubhouse, and boathouses. The *Advertiser-Gleam* estimated that 4,000 attended the opening. The Alabama Warrior Ski Club performed for the crowd. (Marshall County Archives.)

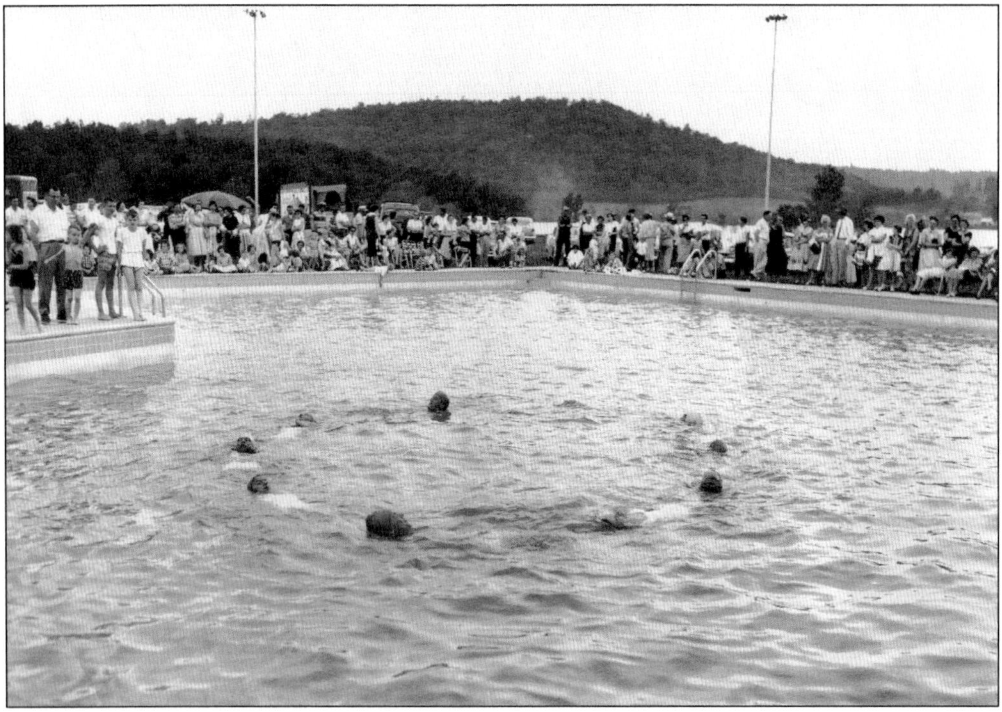

This is the pool at Val Monte Shores, which opened in Guntersville in 1958. The president of Val Monte was Cullen Goss, and the golf professional was Bert Wilde. That same year, a Val Monte women's golf association formed, and the first officers were president Arba Mae Hindman (Guntersville), vice president Louise Sahag (Warrenton), and secretary Quida Reynolds (Arab). (Marshall County Archives.)

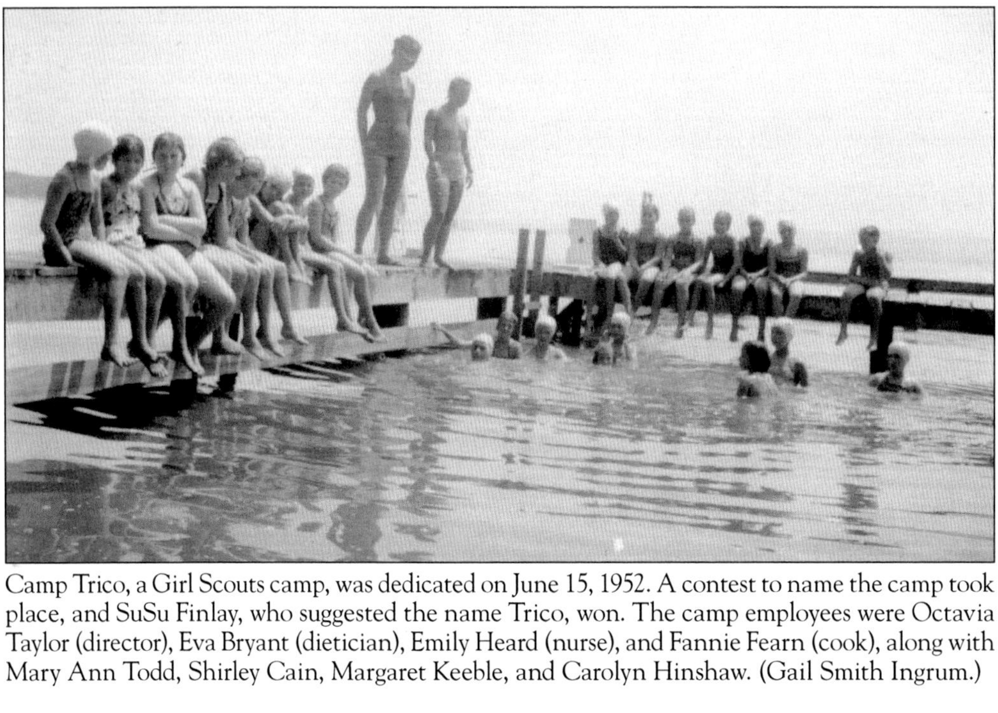

Camp Trico, a Girl Scouts camp, was dedicated on June 15, 1952. A contest to name the camp took place, and SuSu Finlay, who suggested the name Trico, won. The camp employees were Octavia Taylor (director), Eva Bryant (dietician), Emily Heard (nurse), and Fannie Fearn (cook), along with Mary Ann Todd, Shirley Cain, Margaret Keeble, and Carolyn Hinshaw. (Gail Smith Ingrum.)

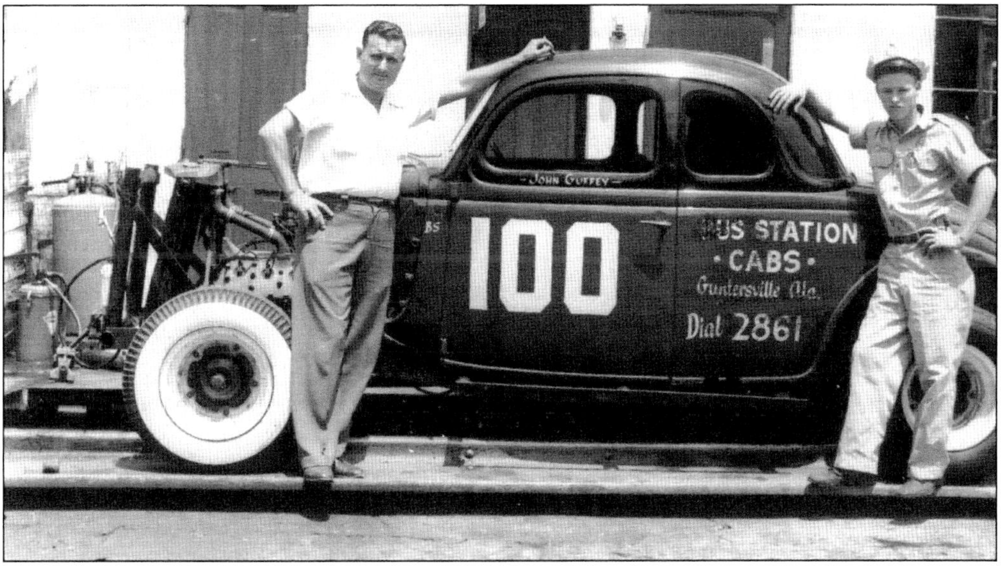

Owners Joe Carter (left) and John H. Guffey are shown in August 1952 with their race car. Every Thursday night, stock car races were held at the Guntersville Speedway. There were seven monetary prizes, and the first-place winner received $500. Among locals who owned stock cars were Melvin Rains, E.B. Hubbard, Buel Locklear, Howard Powell, and Arlis Beal. (Larry Smith.)

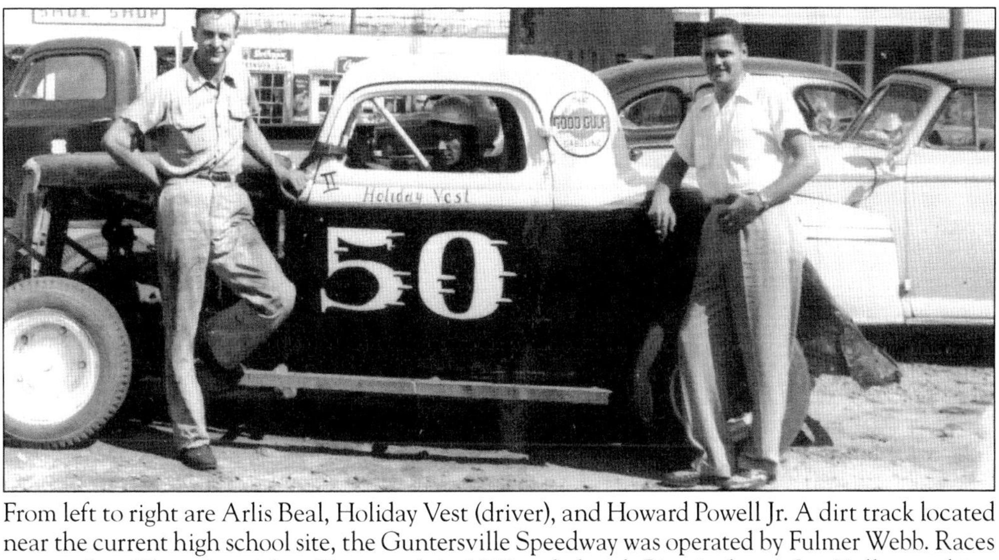

From left to right are Arlis Beal, Holiday Vest (driver), and Howard Powell Jr. A dirt track located near the current high school site, the Guntersville Speedway was operated by Fulmer Webb. Races occurred on Thursday nights. One wreck in 1952 ended with Birmingham's Joe Holley crashing into the lake. Holley was shaken but unscathed. (Larry Smith.)

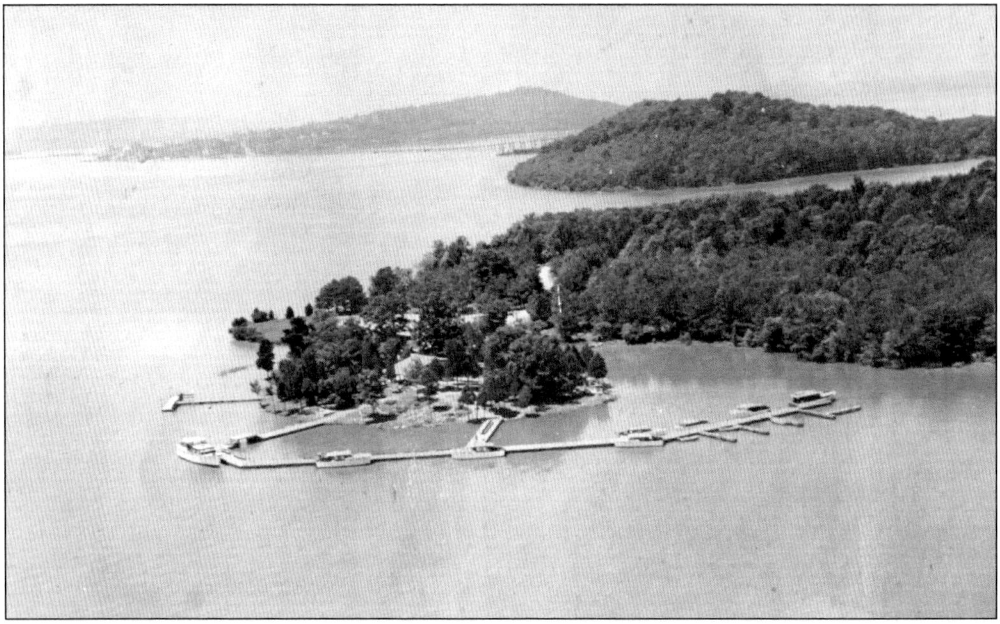

This is the Guntersville Yacht Club around the 1950s. The club was formed in March 1939, and its founding members were Nell Mitchell, Mary Alice Long, Martha Bradford, Dorris Harris, Ann Alves, Martha Sanford, Martha McKee, Willie Ruth Eubanks, Jimmie Land, Walter Posey, Sloppy Starnes, Grady Hipp, Tom Glover Jr., Red White, Chubby Davis, Ruble Bobo, Freelon Manning, and Rip Coplin. (Mike Jones.)

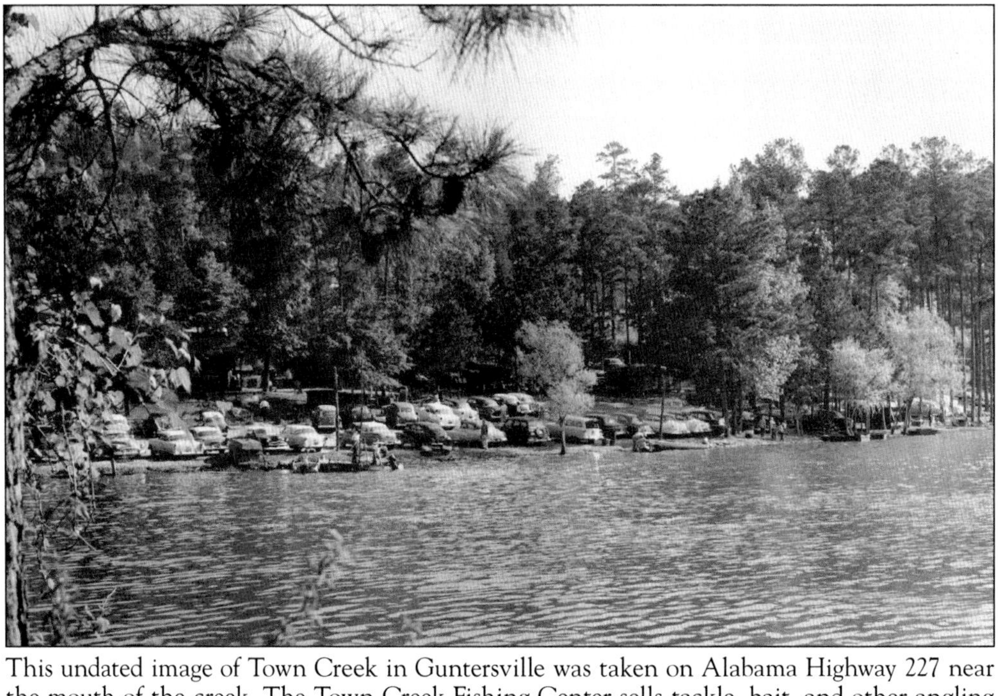

This undated image of Town Creek in Guntersville was taken on Alabama Highway 227 near the mouth of the creek. The Town Creek Fishing Center sells tackle, bait, and other angling necessities. It also rents pontoon and bass boats, as well as canoes and flat bottoms. It boasts a nice campground. (Guntersville Historical Society.)

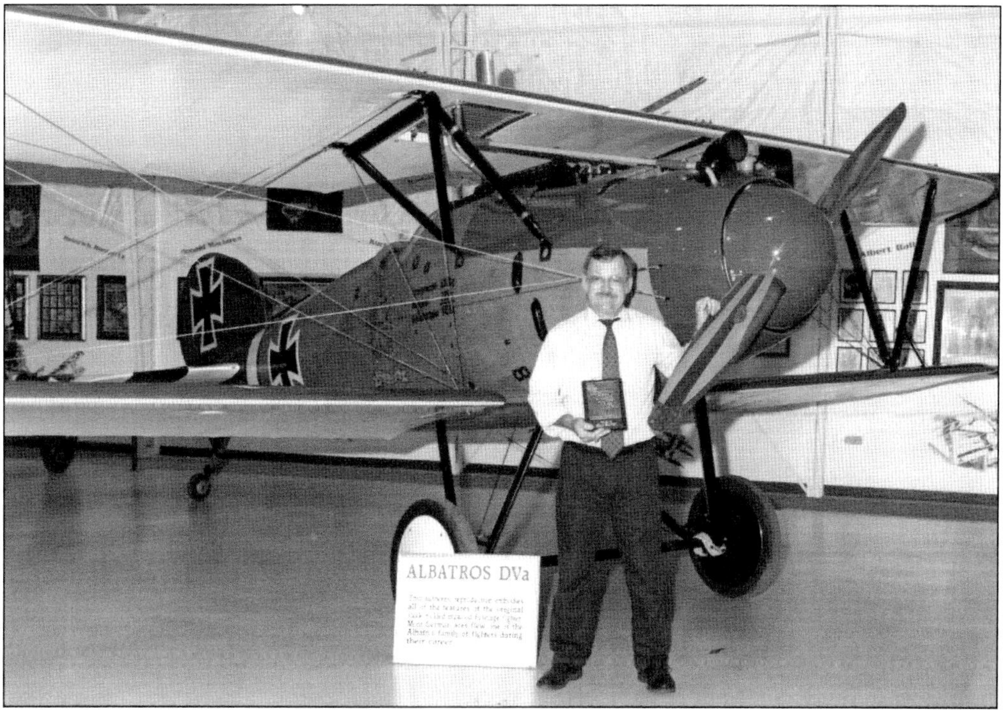

Frank Ryder opened a World War I replica fighter museum in Guntersville in 1988. It had 40 replicas and a variety of war-related antiques. Originally from Indiana, Ryder moved to Arab in 1978 and opened Ryder International. Tragically, in 1994, while planning a move to Guntersville, he, his wife, Carolyn, and son, Scott, were killed in a plane crash. (*Advertiser-Gleam.*)

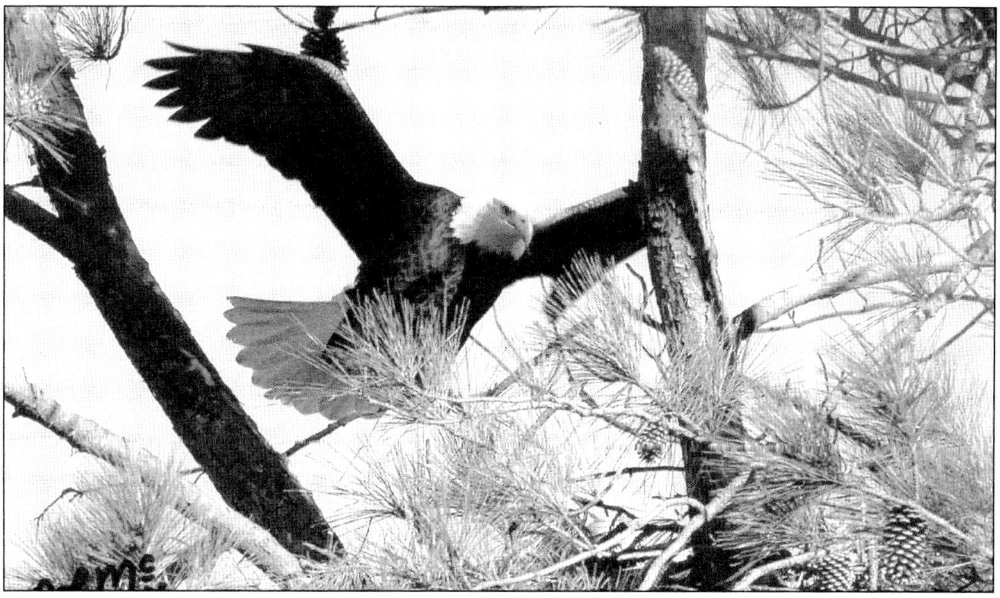

The area below the Tennessee Valley Authority Guntersville Dam is a popular bald eagle nesting area. In 2012, one set of bald eagles, dubbed Barney and Thelma Lou, attracted much attention with their three chicks. At that time, there were roughly 75 bald eagles in the Guntersville area and 20 nests. (*Advertiser-Gleam.*)

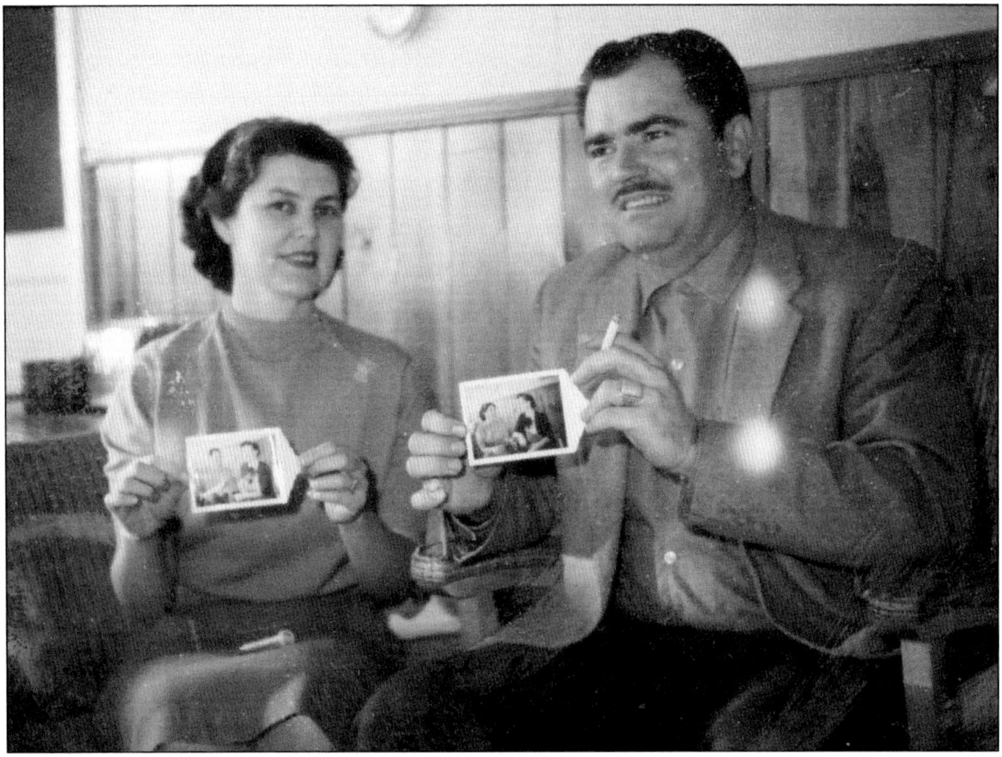

Ida Will Willis Smith (left) and Jay Gurley display photographs taken with her new Polaroid camera. Gurley, a photographer by profession, purchased an enormous cave in Grant, Marshall County, in 1952, named it Cathedral Caverns, and opened it to the public in 1955. It quickly became one of the most popular tourist attractions in Alabama. (Gail Smith Ingrum.)

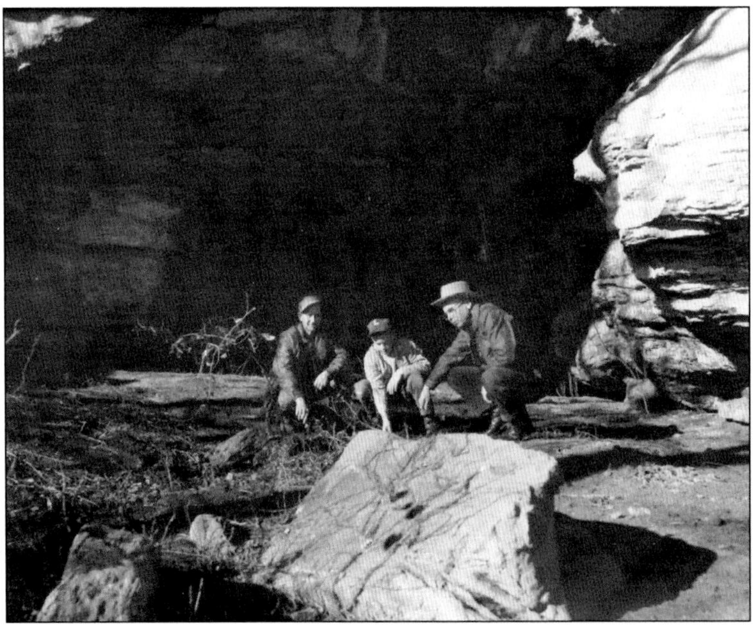

From left to right are John D. Gilbreath, unidentified, and Ed Mahan. Mahan performed extensive excavations in caves throughout the area. One of his favorites was Cathedral Caverns. Over the years, he found many Native American artifacts, primarily in the entrance area. (Nancy Gilbreath Graham.)

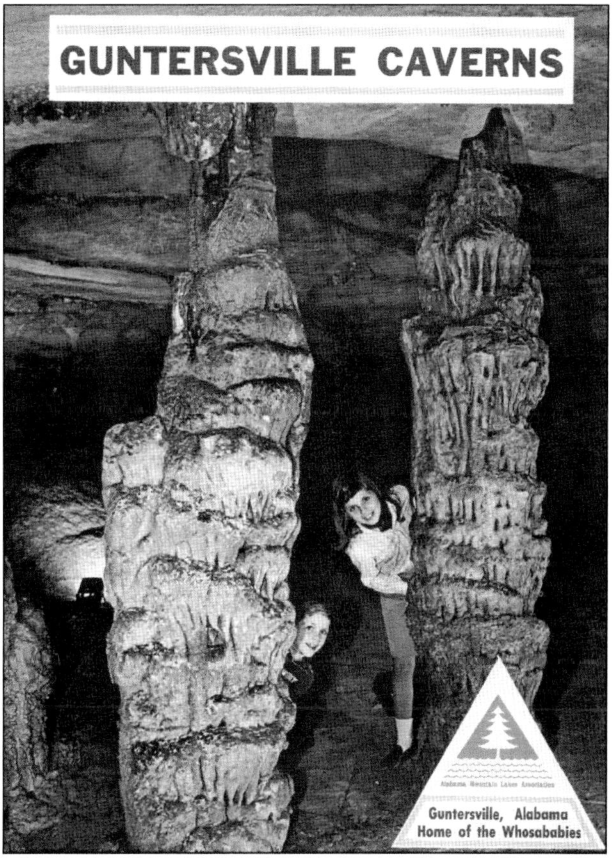

Known for colorful formations and sea fossils, Guntersville Caverns was opened by Joe and Gwen Reeves in 1958. Guntersville Caverns' main attractions were the Onyx Pathway, the Wishing Well, the Twin Columns (shown), the Lion's Cage, the Balanced Rock, the Blueberry Rock, and the Whosababies sandstone formations. This tourist attraction closed in the early 1970s. (David Jones.)

In this 1990s photograph are, from left to right, Howard Hawk (then Alabama House member), June Fricks (then marketing manager of Lake Guntersville State Park), Tom Bevill (then US representative), and unidentified. Fricks, who spent almost 30 years at the park, was also a member of the Marshall County Tourism Board. (Lake Guntersville State Park.)

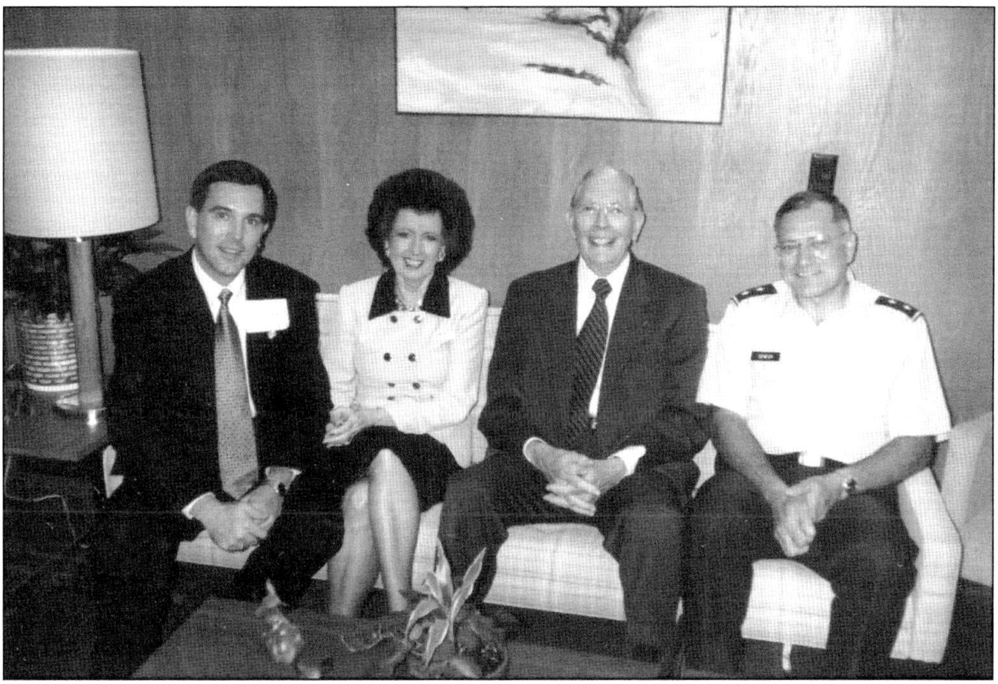

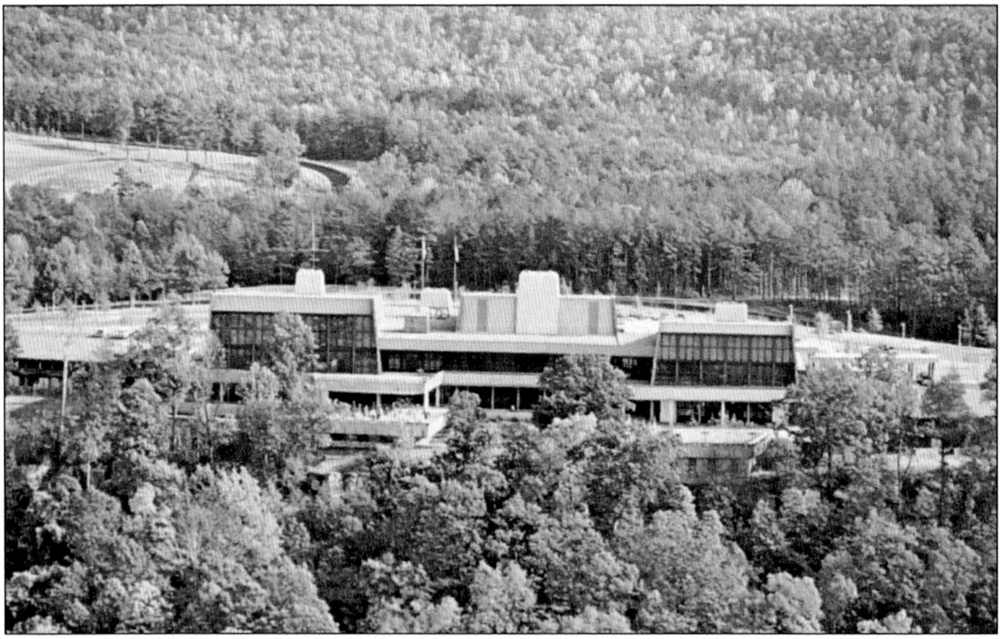

This is a photograph of the lodge at Lake Guntersville State Park. Nestled in the trees atop a mountain, it has glorious views of the lake below. Sunrise and sunset are especially breathtaking. Many hiking trails and zip lines await guests. The lodge accommodations are lush, and the restaurant is exceptional. (Lake Guntersville State Park.)

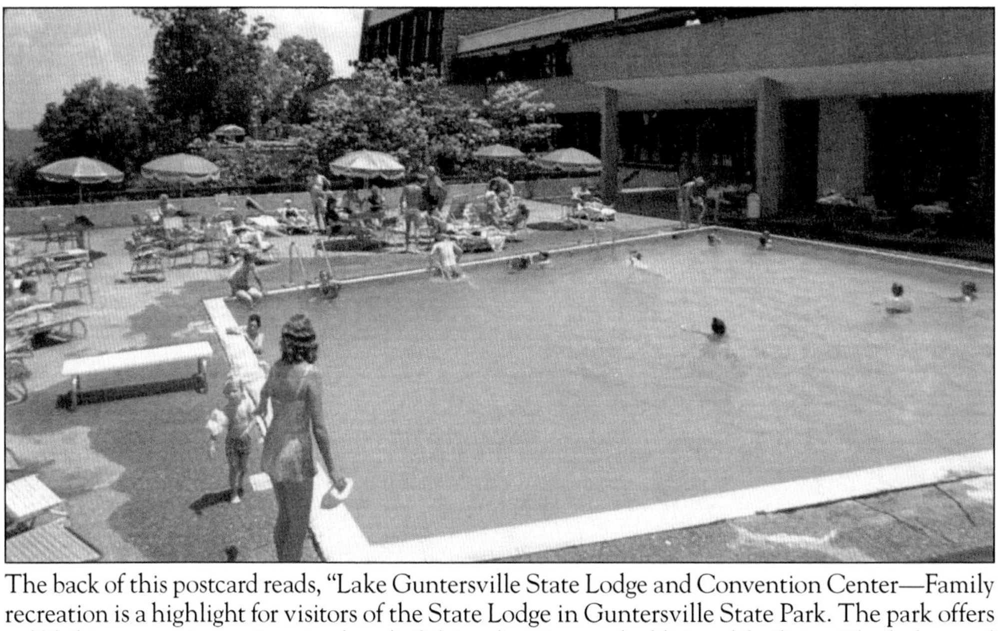

The back of this postcard reads, "Lake Guntersville State Lodge and Convention Center—Family recreation is a highlight for visitors of the State Lodge in Guntersville State Park. The park offers golf, hiking, camping, swimming beach, fishing, boating, and additional facilities. The lodge pool is always active during warm summer days with children and parents enjoying the sunshine and cool water." (Lake Guntersville State Park.)

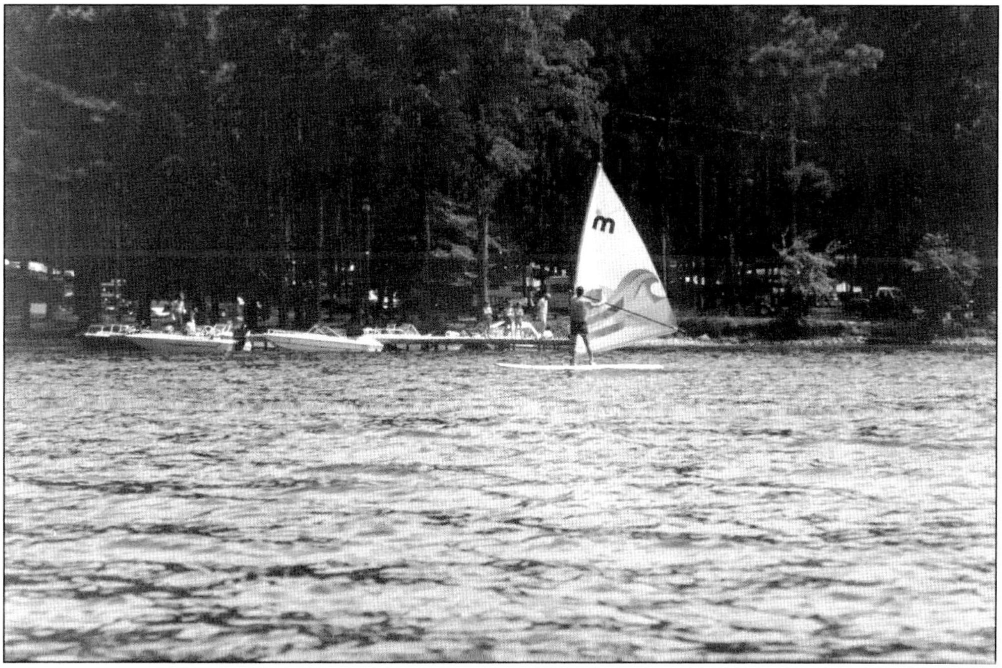

This is an undated image of the campground at Lake Guntersville State Park. Windsurfing, skiing, canoeing, kayaking, jet skiing, and tubing are all popular forms of entertainment on the lake. In addition to the beach at the state park, there is one on Sunset Drive in Guntersville. (Lake Guntersville State Park.)

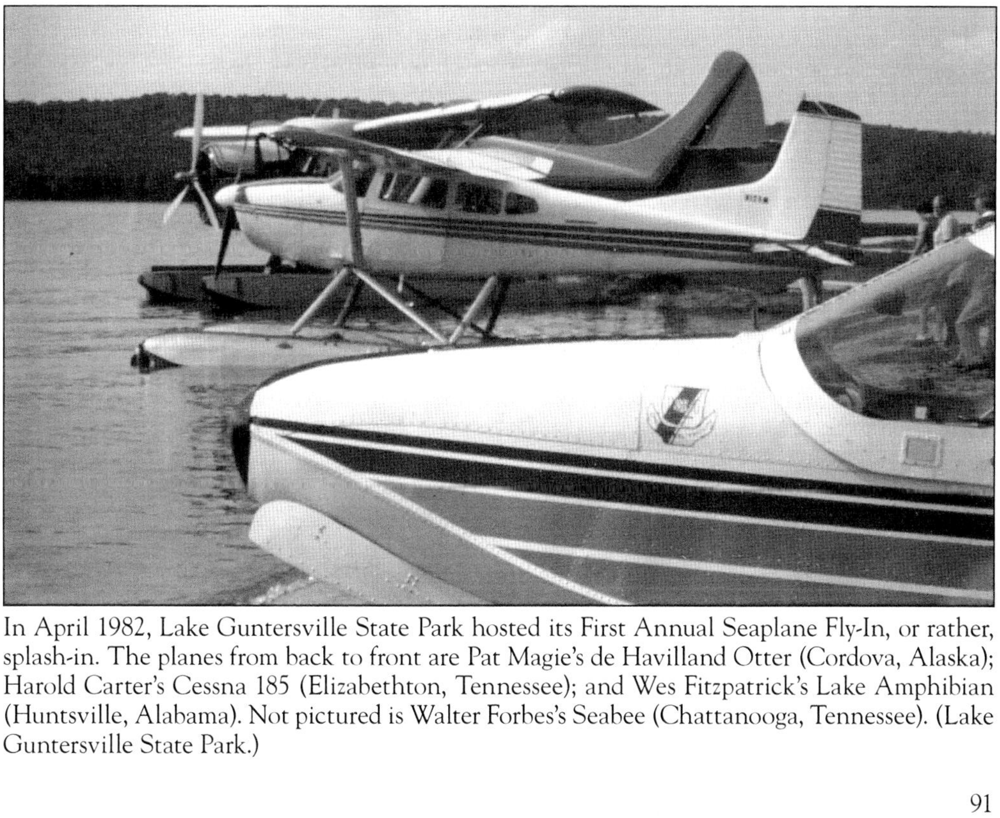

In April 1982, Lake Guntersville State Park hosted its First Annual Seaplane Fly-In, or rather, splash-in. The planes from back to front are Pat Magie's de Havilland Otter (Cordova, Alaska); Harold Carter's Cessna 185 (Elizabethton, Tennessee); and Wes Fitzpatrick's Lake Amphibian (Huntsville, Alabama). Not pictured is Walter Forbes's Seabee (Chattanooga, Tennessee). (Lake Guntersville State Park.)

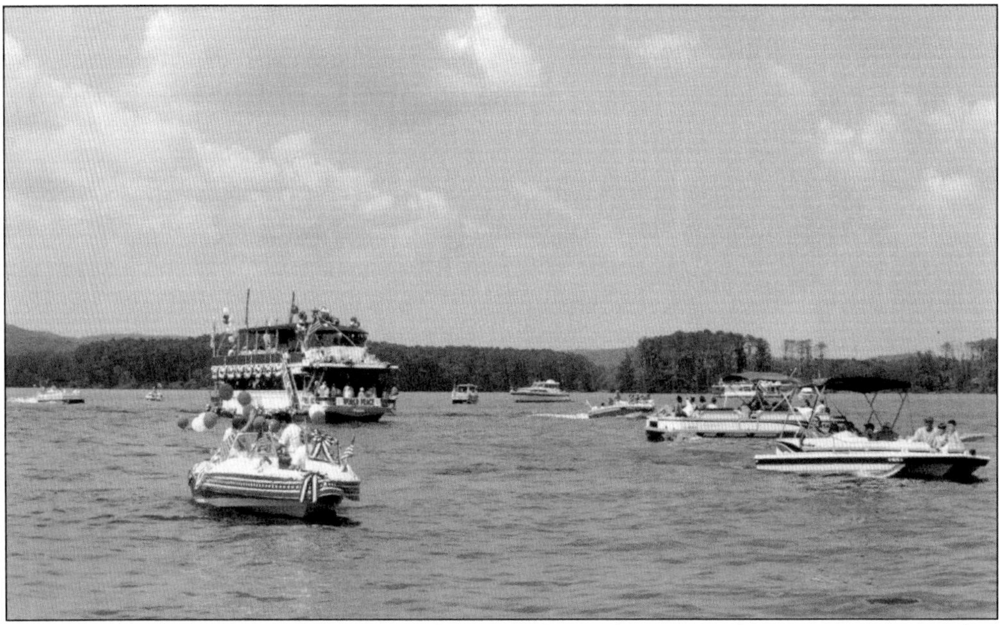

Patriotic fervor embraced Guntersville in this image from July 4, 1999. The city commemorated its sesquicentennial (1848–1998) with multiple events. A stern-wheeler float represented Guntersville in the inaugural parade of Gov. Don Siegelman. Ambassadors were the second-grade students, who all journeyed to Montgomery for the inauguration. (Guntersville City Hall.)

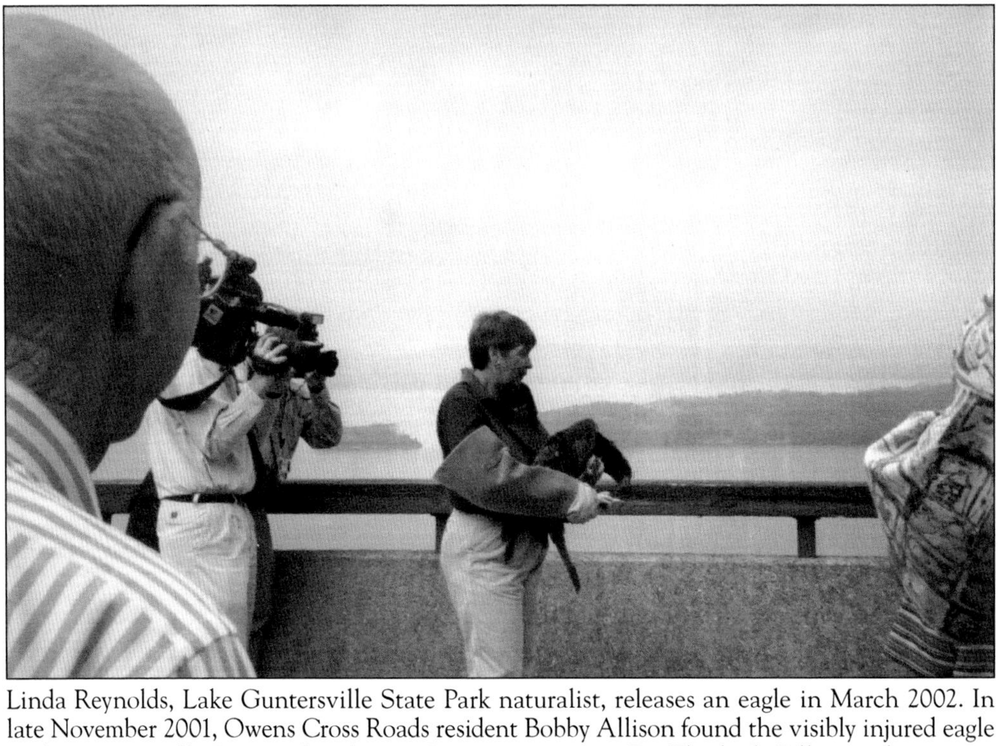

Linda Reynolds, Lake Guntersville State Park naturalist, releases an eagle in March 2002. In late November 2001, Owens Cross Roads resident Bobby Allison found the visibly injured eagle at the Guntersville Dam and took it to Grant veterinarian Dr. Elizabeth Billings, who in turn transported it to Auburn University, where it was rehabilitated. (Lake Guntersville State Park.)

Four

SCENES AND PERSONALITIES

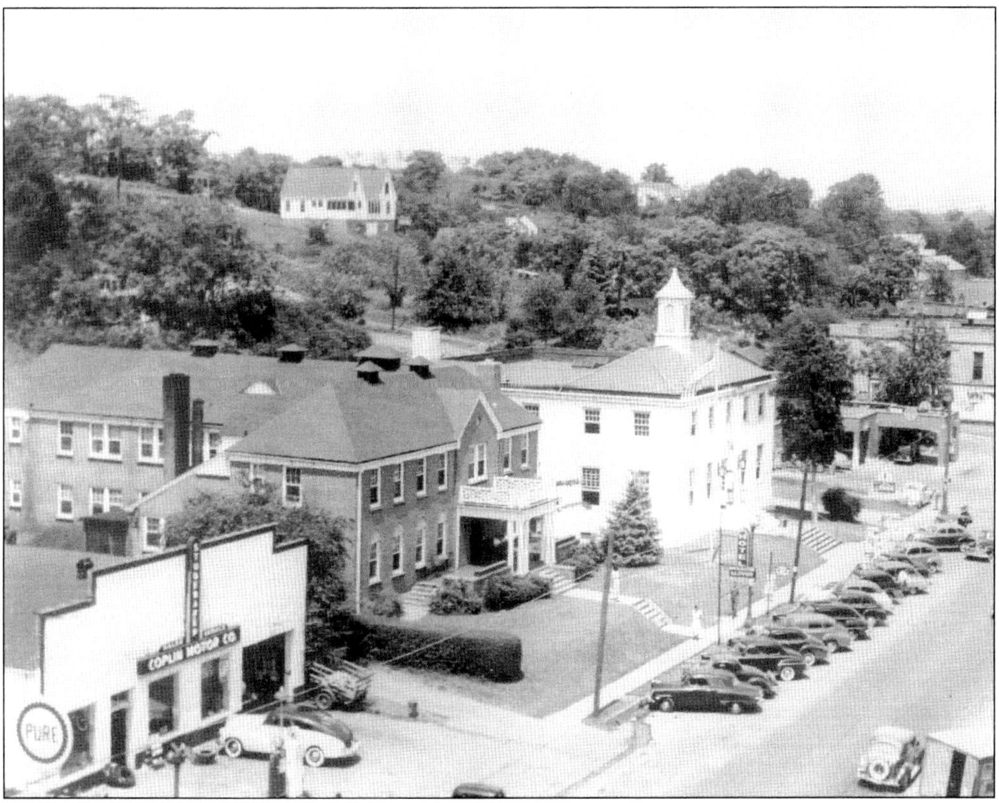

This is a 1940s aerial view of downtown Guntersville. The building on the far left is the Coplin Motor Company. The building second from left is the Glover Hotel. The building third from left is the old post office. Note the houses dotting the hill in the background. (Marshall County Archives.)

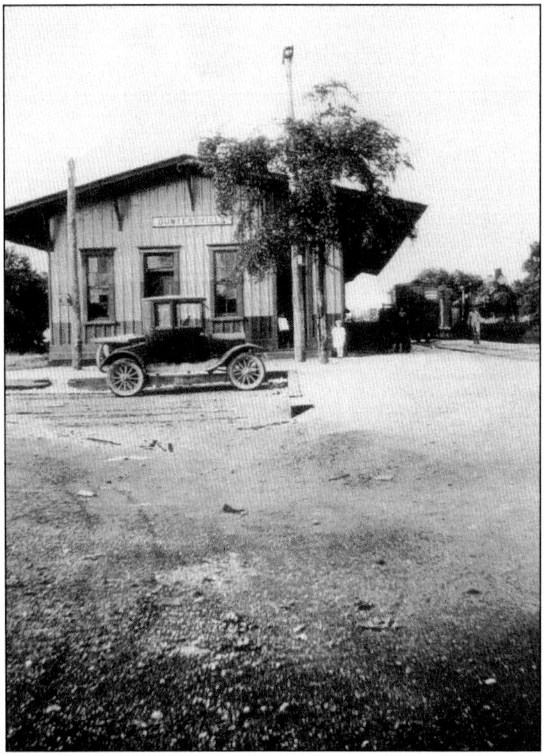

This undated photograph shows the Guntersville Depot. Built in 1892, it was restored by the Guntersville Historical Society beginning in 1996 and opened in 2000 as the Guntersville Railroad Depot Museum. The depot is the subject of a lovely watercolor print by the late Mildred Meyer. (Guntersville Historical Society.)

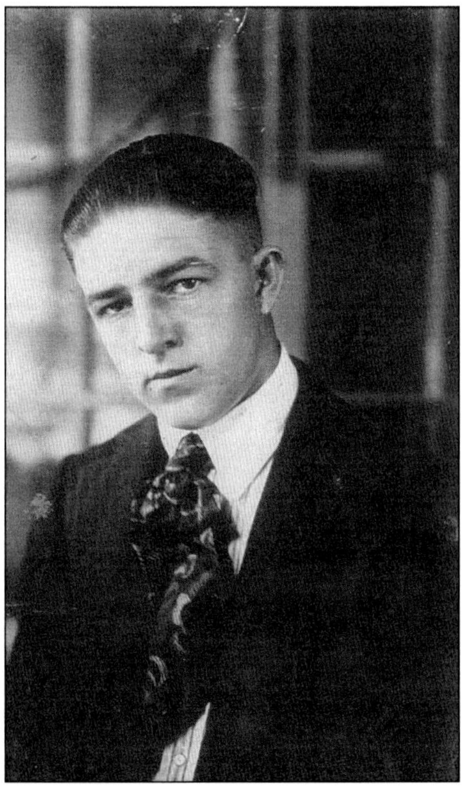

Born in Guntersville in 1900, William Nabors left the area in 1919 and traveled the country as a hobo. He eventually settled in Greenwich Village, New York City, where he gained attention as a writer, poet, and journalist. His noteworthy friends included but were not limited to Maxwell Bodenheim, Vachel Lindsay, Edwin Markham, "Hobo King" Dan O'Brien, and "Hobo Queen" Boxcar Betty. (Authors' collection.)

Major excitement gripped Guntersville when electrical power became accessible in homes and businesses. Rural electrification enhanced the lives of the members of the community and improved economic development. After 1939, electrical power became the norm instead of the exception. (Larry Smith.)

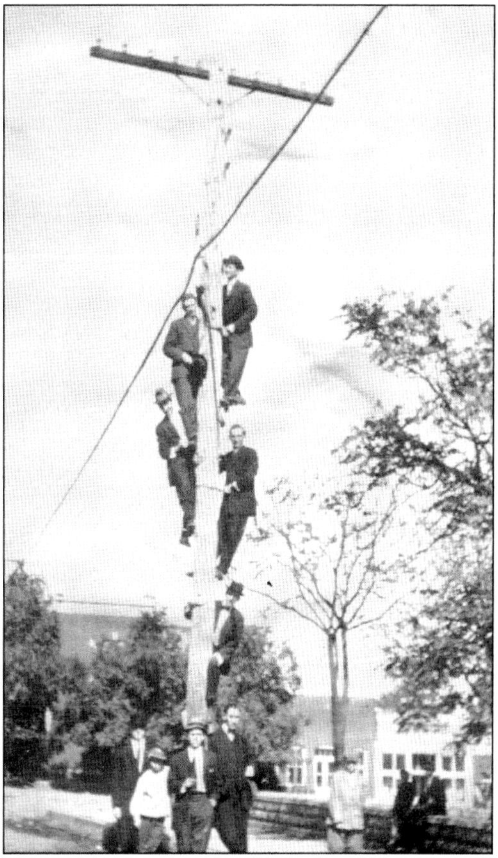

Jack's Café in Guntersville was opened in 1946 by Warner Jackson and later moved. In 1956, it was sold to J.B. and Monroe McKinney. When Monroe died, Jackson, who by that time operated Mrs. Jackson's Steakhouse, repurchased the café. In 1967, it was sold to Otto Smallwood, who two years later sold it Pete Johnson; Johnson renamed the café Annie's Country Kitchen. (Nancy Gilbreath Graham.)

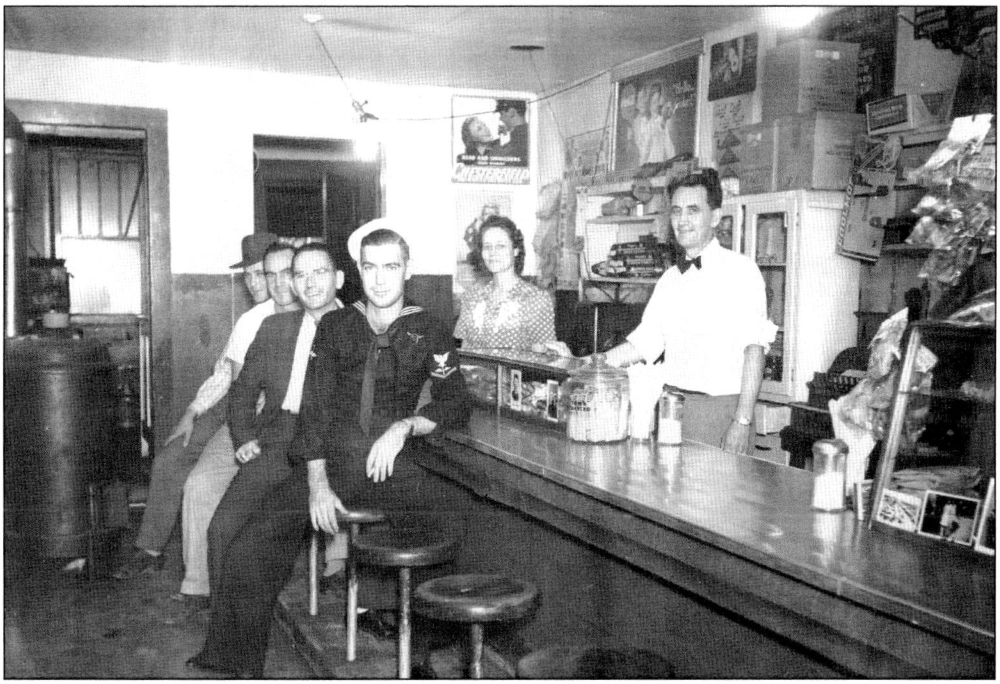

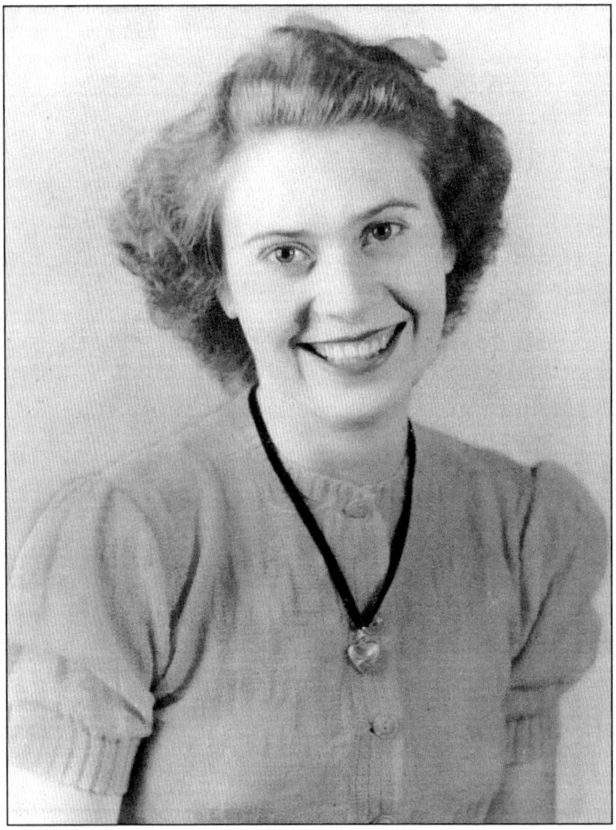

Cora Cooley, daughter of Malinda and Bid Cooley, graduated from Marshall County High School in 1941. She taught school during World War II, worked in a defense plant, and married Kenneth Gross in 1944. They later farmed on Georgia Mountain and had children, Barbara and Ken. Cora worked at Blue Bell, Lee Factory, and Ryder International. In her retirement, she pampered her granddaughters, Jennifer Gross and Whitney Snow. (Authors' collection.)

These are veterans who returned from World War II and graduated from Marshall County High School in 1947. From left to right are (first row) J.R. Williams (teacher), J.P. Green, Norman Propes, Pete Duncan, and Joe Woods; (second row) Howard Powell Jr., Joe Birdsong, Edward Rollings, Jack Pritchett, and T.S. Wiles. (Guntersville Museum.)

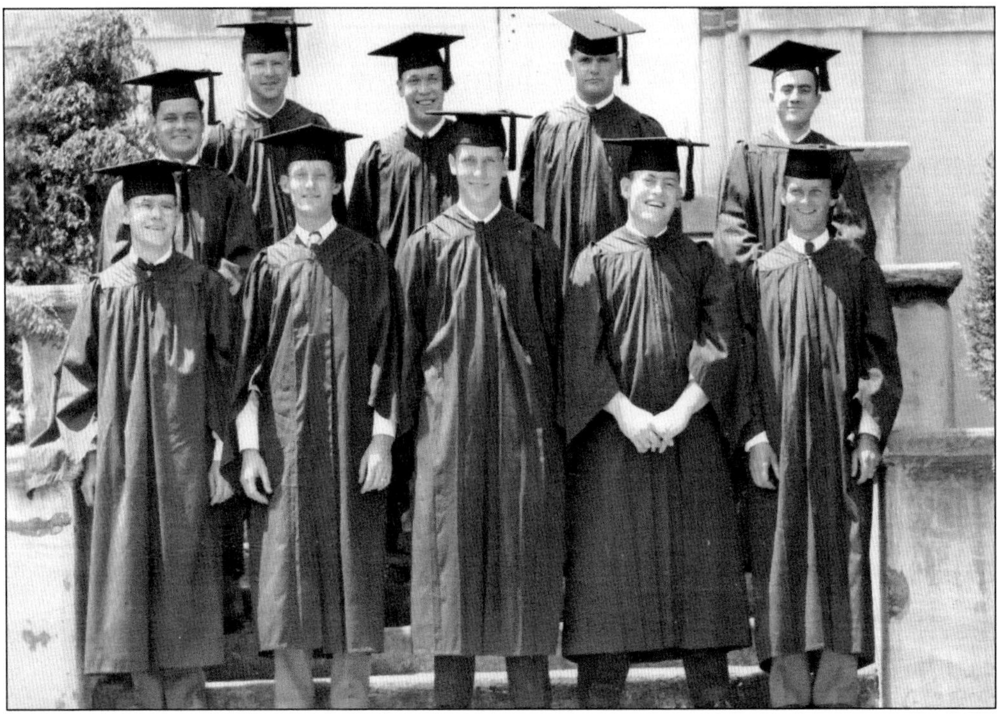

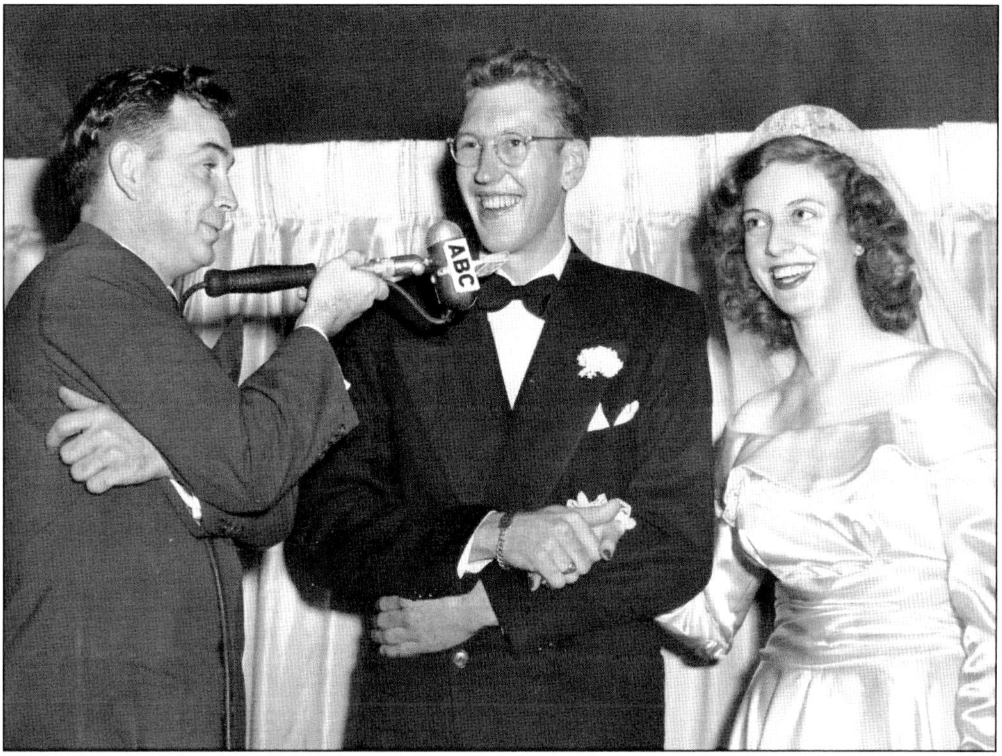

On March 24, 1949, John Fricke and Roberta Allison got married on the *Bride and Groom* radio program in Hollywood, California. The couple talked of their first date on Reservoir Hill and of the beauty of Guntersville. For appearing on the show, the couple received a camera, a washing machine, a phonograph, a wedding album, and a honeymoon at the Flamingo Hotel in Las Vegas. (Marshall County Archives.)

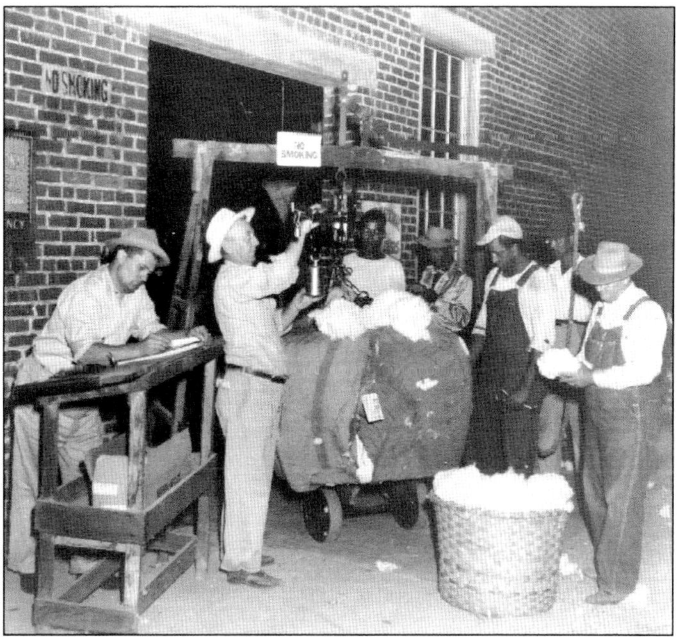

Harvey D. Johnson (far left), Dayton Gilbreath (second from left), and Fred Hawk (far right) are shown weighing cotton at the Gilbreath and Hawk Cotton Warehouse. The other individuals in the photograph are unidentified. Johnson, Gilbreath, and Hawk were all very active in civic and business affairs. (Marshall County Archives.)

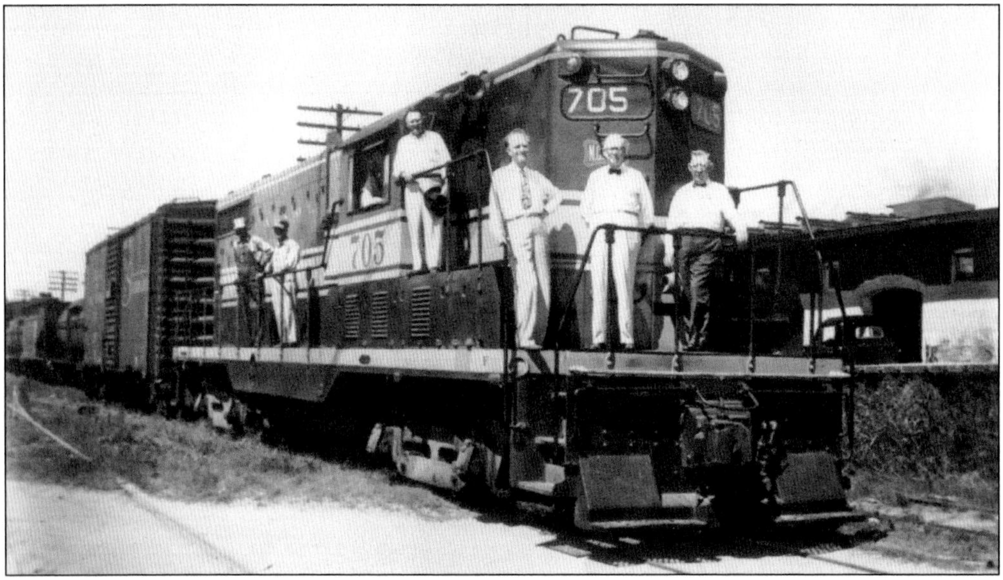

Taken by Robert O. Johnson on September 23, 1950, this is a photograph of the first diesel engine used by the Nashville, Chattanooga & St. Louis Railway on the Tennessee & Coosa Branch. In no particular order are A.M. Morgan (conductor), A.F. Jones (station agent, Albertville), E.W. Crabtree (trainmaster), and J.W. Tucker (division superintendent). (Guntersville Historical Society.)

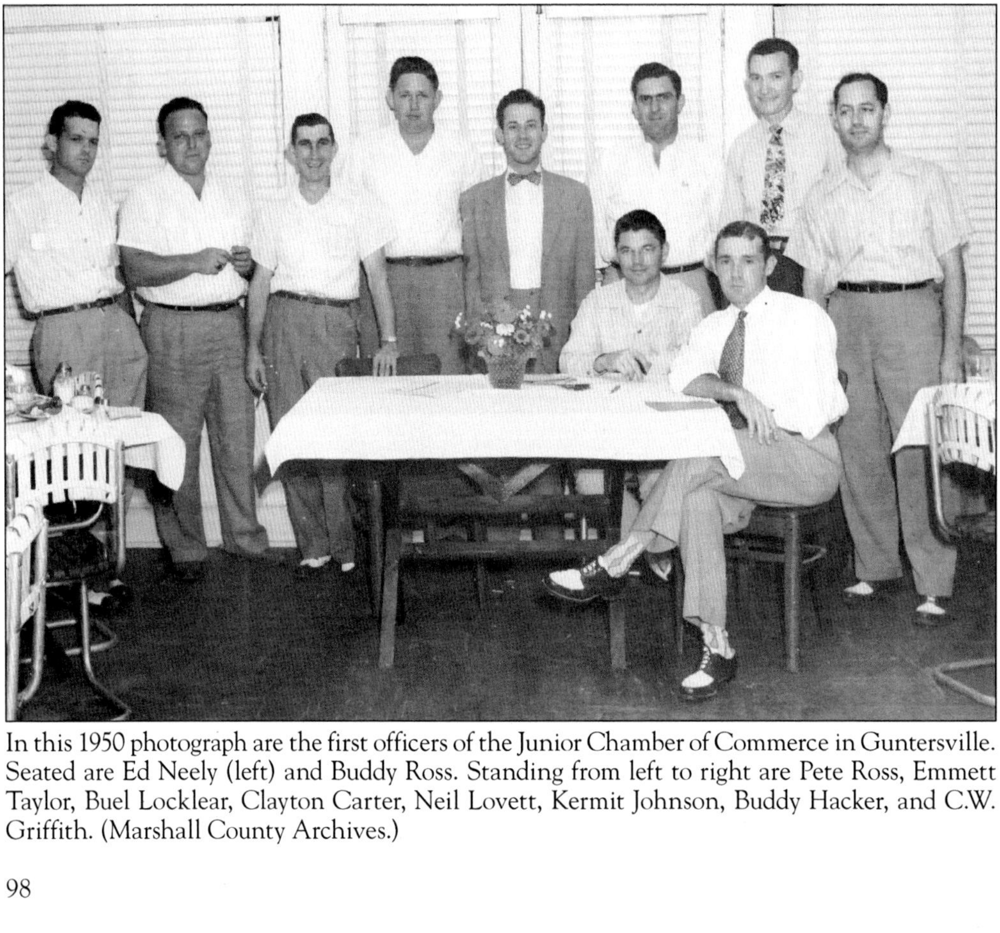

In this 1950 photograph are the first officers of the Junior Chamber of Commerce in Guntersville. Seated are Ed Neely (left) and Buddy Ross. Standing from left to right are Pete Ross, Emmett Taylor, Buel Locklear, Clayton Carter, Neil Lovett, Kermit Johnson, Buddy Hacker, and C.W. Griffith. (Marshall County Archives.)

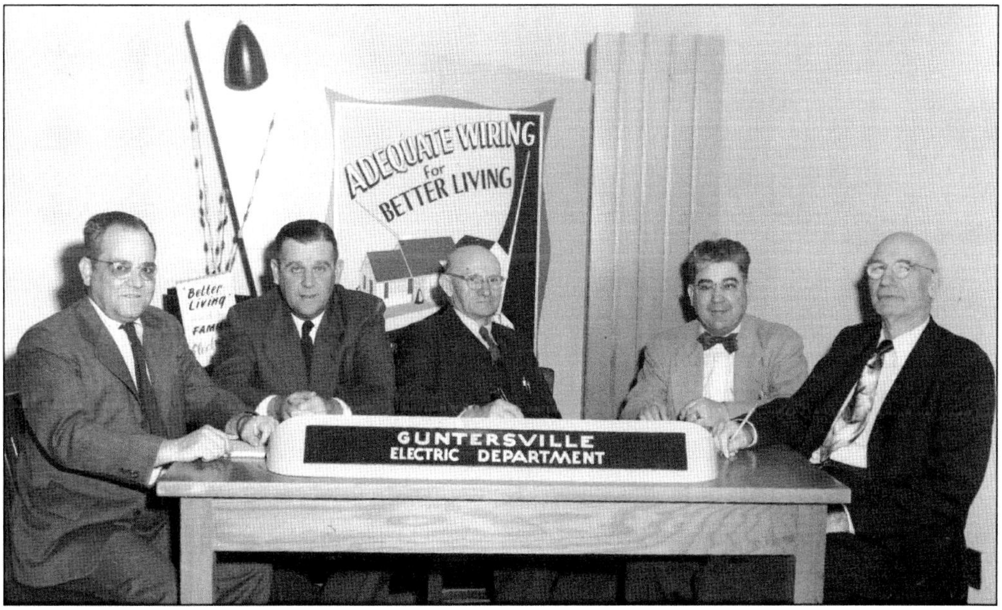

This is the 1952 Electric Board in Guntersville. From left to right are John H. Carter (manager), Timmons Jordan, Paul W. Stockton, John T. Sulzby, and E.H. Couch. Employees were Carter (manager), M.P. Marsh (line foreman), Johnnie Smith (lineman), Holland Duvall (helper), Jean Benefield (bookkeeper), George Nix (assistant bookkeeper), J.E. Brown (meter reader), R.L. Chandler (meter reader), and Roy Alexander (lineman helper). (Marshall County Archives.)

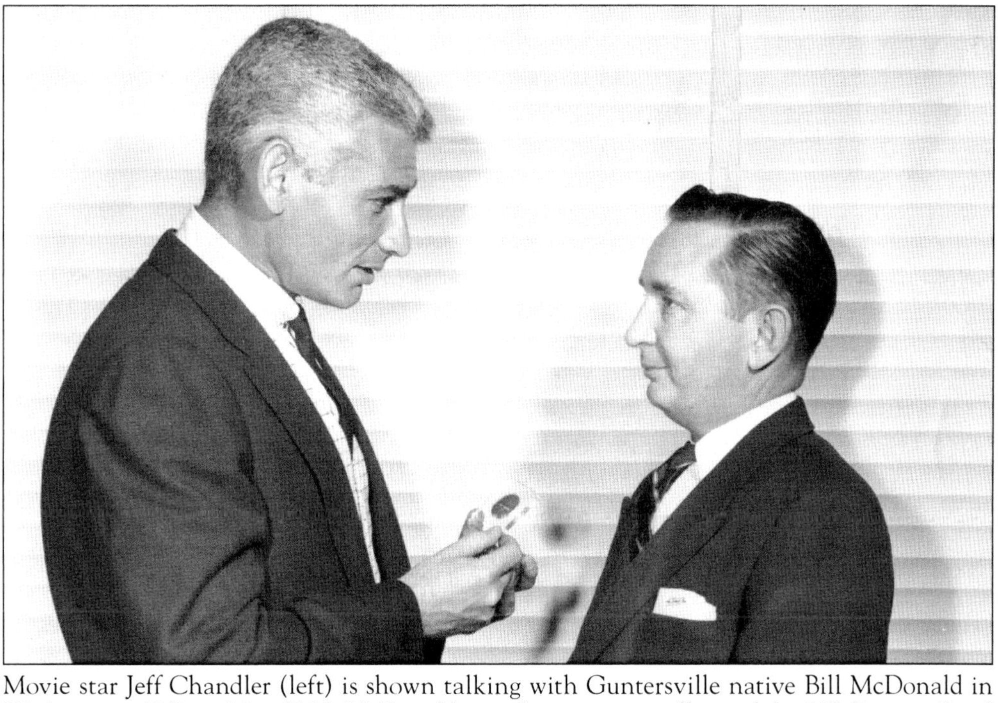

Movie star Jeff Chandler (left) is shown talking with Guntersville native Bill McDonald in Washington, DC, in May 1956. McDonald was the executive officer of the US Savings Bond Division in the nation's capital and met many other celebrities, like Barbara Stanwyck. He married Guntersville girl Viola Simms. (Marshall County Archives.)

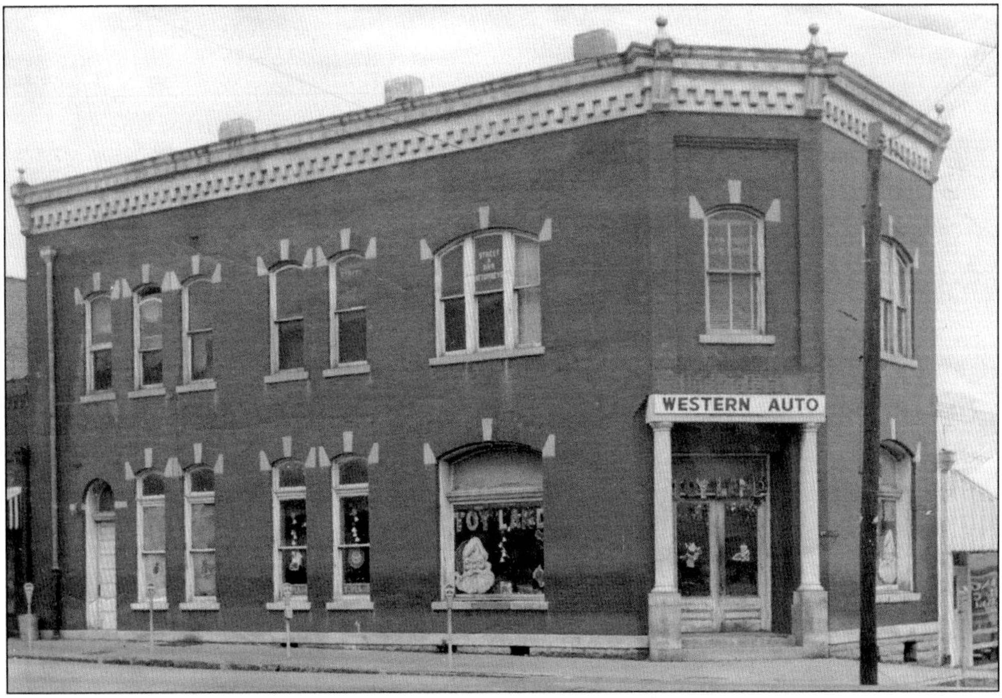

In 1906, the Bank of Guntersville completed a structure with elaborate interiors at the corner of Gunter Avenue and Taylor Street. In its heyday, deposits exceeded $100,000. In 1916, the financial institution closed because of troubled accounting. The building was acquired by the Citizens Bank and was later rented by Western Auto. It is now the Corner Market. (Larry Smith.)

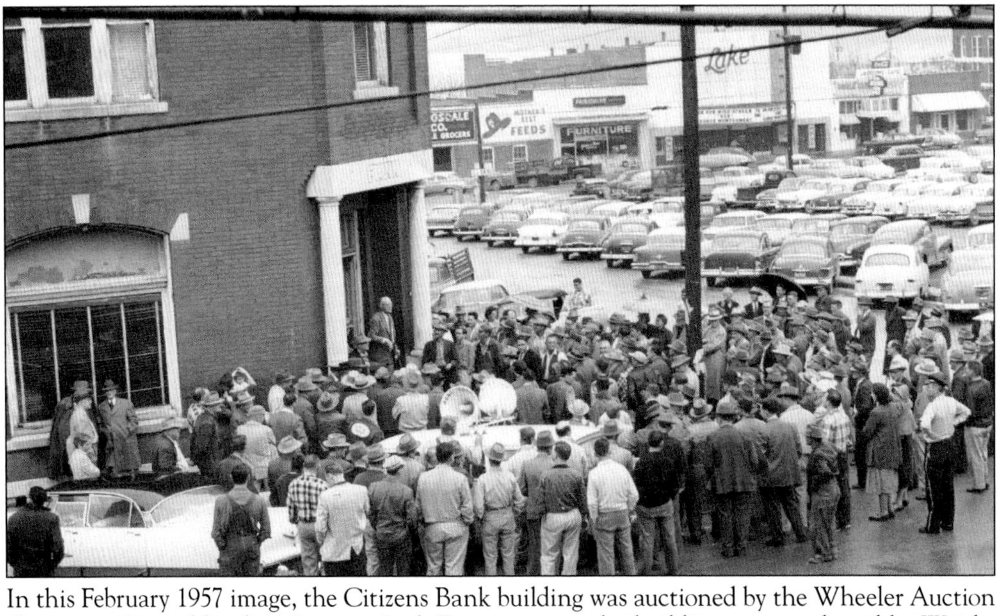

In this February 1957 image, the Citizens Bank building was auctioned by the Wheeler Auction Company. Owned by the Margaret Lusk Farrow estate, the building was purchased by Wright Ross for $21,000. The *Advertiser-Gleam* called it "the highest price per square foot ever paid for property in Guntersville." The Lake Theatre is visible in the background. (Guntersville Historical Society.)

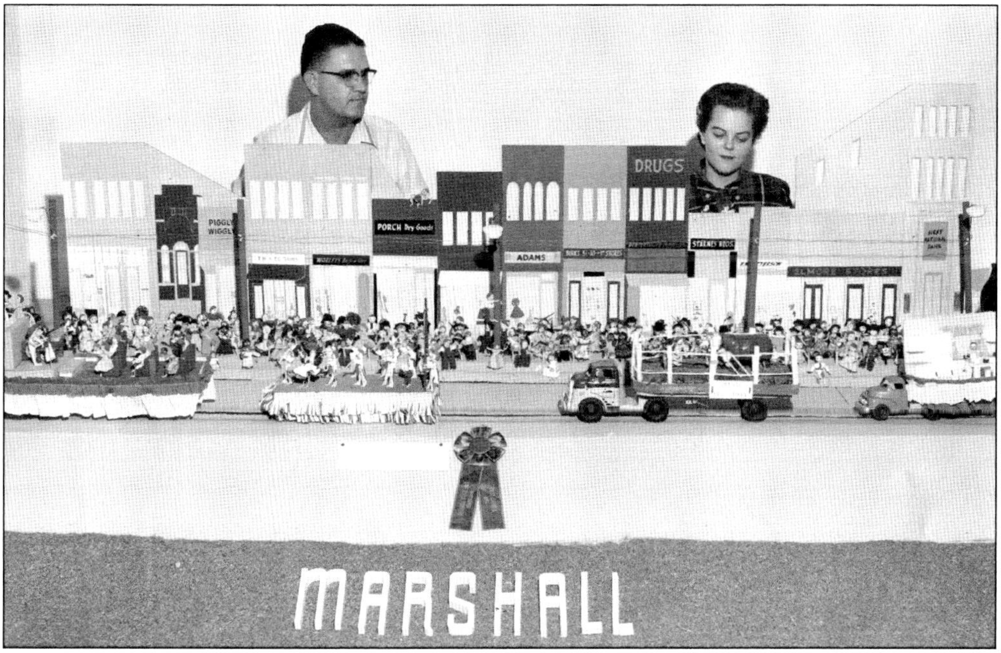

This is an undated photograph of an impressive model of Gunter Avenue. The shops shown are Piggly Wiggly, TM&TG Rains, Worley's Bargain Store, Porch Dry Goods, Adams, Burk's 5¢-10¢-$1.00 Stores, Guntersville Pharmacy, Starnes Bros., F.W. Patterson, Elmore Stores, and the First National Bank. (Marshall County Archives.)

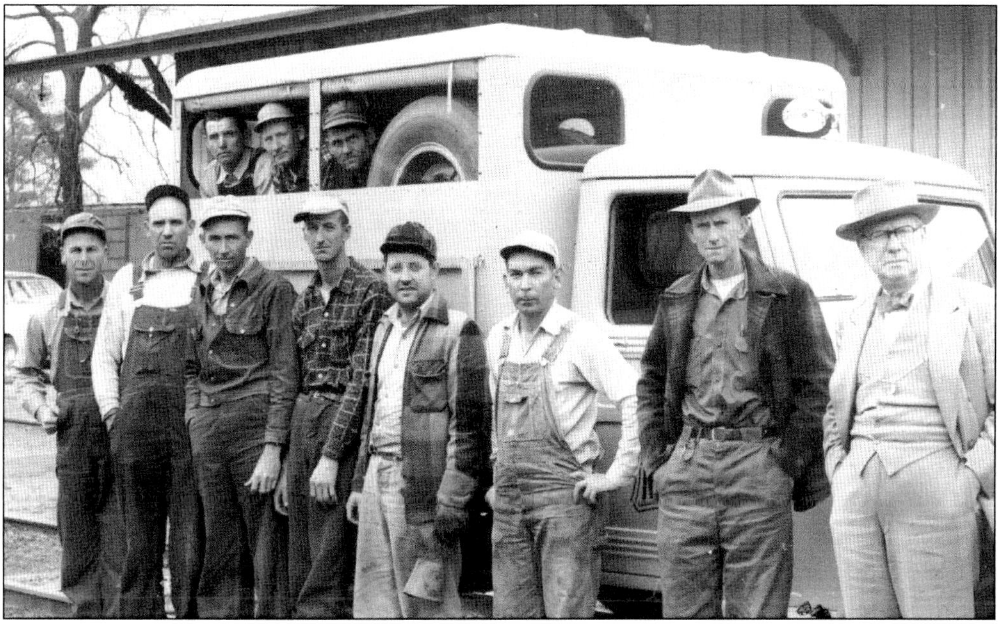

In this undated photograph, Nashville, Chattanooga & St. Louis Railway section hands are pictured with a rail/highway motorcar. From left to right in the car are unidentified, Robert McKay, and Joe Noogin. Standing, from left to right, are Earl Holmes, J.H. James, Dick Burns, unidentified, ? Simmons, R.T. Hyatt, R.E. Morehead, and E.W. Crabtree (trainmaster). (Marshall County Archives.)

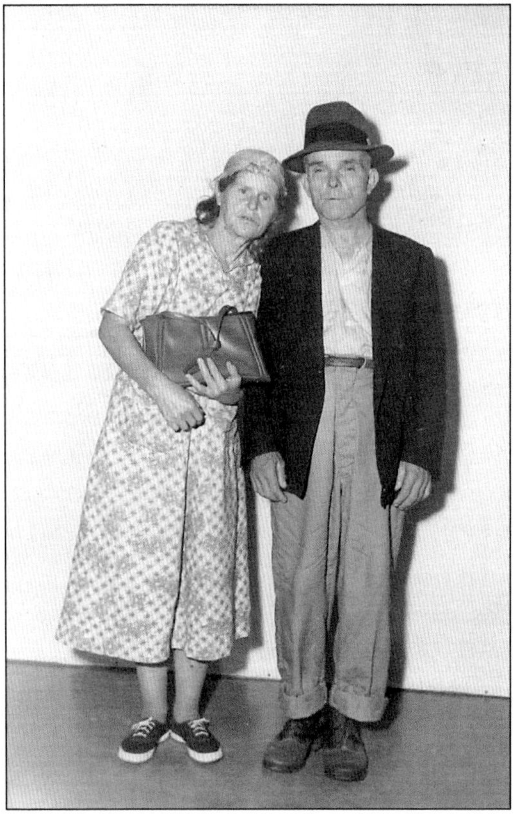

Shown are eccentrics Arthur P. "Stocklaw" Johnson and his wife, Dora. From the 1930s until his death in 1955, they lived in Polecat Hollow and earned money selling things like kindling and poke salat. They solicited money in exchange for singing (and not singing) and playing records on a portable phonograph. They also charged people to pose with them in photographs. (*Advertiser-Gleam.*)

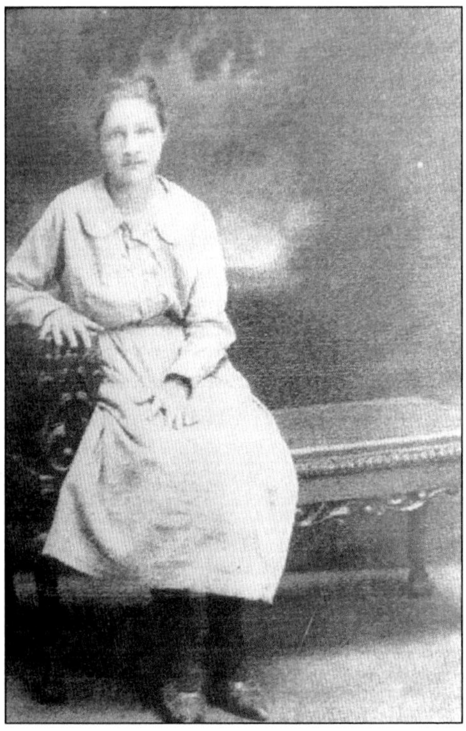

This is Arthur "Stocklaw" Johnson's first wife, Bessie Jane. The daughter of Joseph and Amanda Childress, Bessie married Stocklaw and, in 1920, they had a son named Jasper. She left Stocklaw in 1922 and divorced him in 1925. In 1926, she remarried Stocklaw and had a daughter named Ellie Mae. Bessie died in 1927. (Johnny Simpson.)

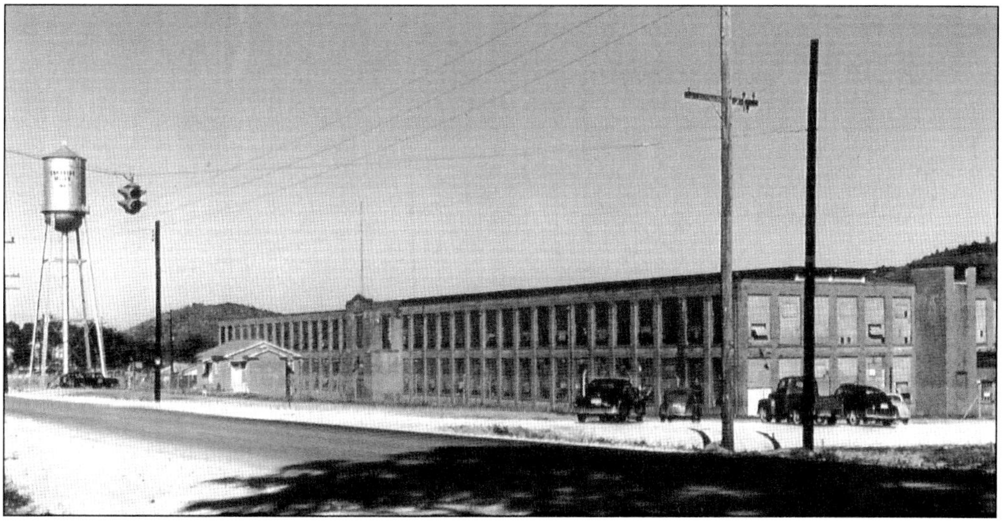

Built by the American Manufacturers Company, the Saratoga Victory Mills opened in 1928. It was sold to Lowenstein & Sons in 1944 and, in 1949, to J.R. Abney, who renamed it Julia Cade Mill. In 1950, it was bought by Hesslein & Company and became Lakeside Mill, which closed in 1957. It is currently the location of Mike's Warehouse, owned by Mike Jones. (Guntersville Museum.)

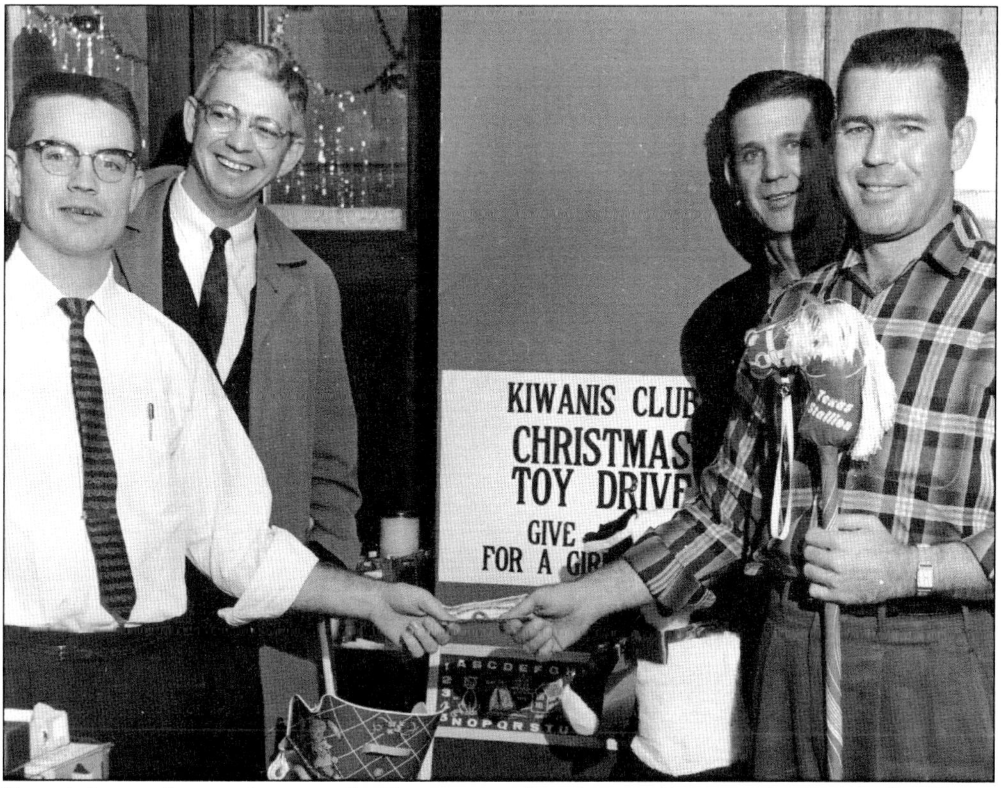

From left to right are Guntersville Kiwanis members Harvey Brown, John Bostwick, John L. Beard, and Grover Burks helping with a Christmas toy drive in 1958. Burks is purchasing a toy. Beard served as chair for the project, while Brown and Bostwick were on the drive committee. (Marshall County Archives.)

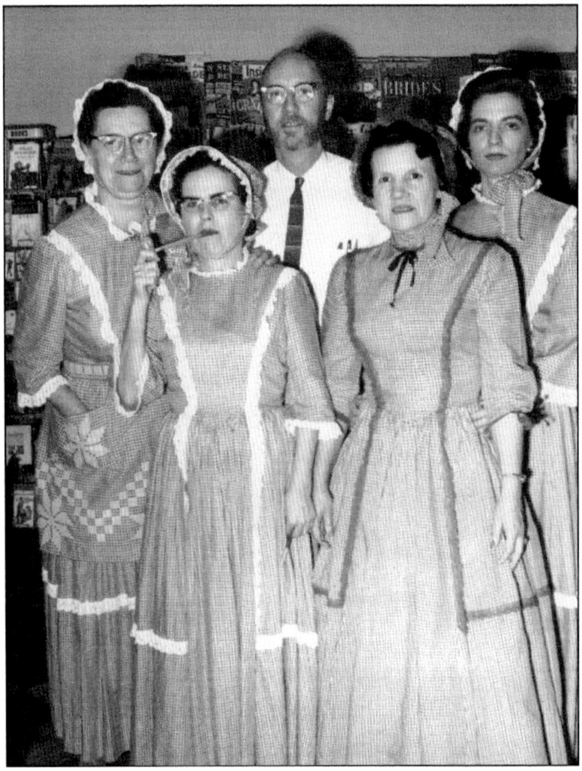

These are employees at the Guntersville Rexall Pharmacy in 1961. From left to right are Neva Bush, Dorothy Webb, Clyde Luttrell, Jennie Patterson, and Virginia Harvell. Not shown are employees Mervin McCormick, Carlisle Hipp, and Mary McDermott, as well as manager Wood Throckmorton. (Marshall County Archives.)

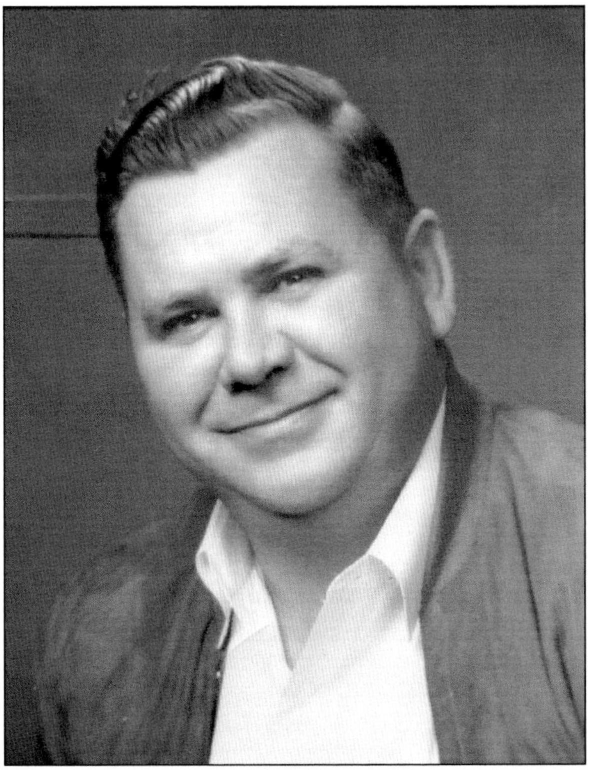

This is Roscoe "Behop" Hopson, who ran the Moonglo Café for 16 years. A resident of Guntersville since the age of 10, he served in World War II and belonged to both the American Legion and Veterans of Foreign Wars. He married Guntersville native Helen Rogers, and they had five daughters: Betty Sue, Juanita, Jan, Linda, and Kriss Lee. (Marshall County Archives.)

Shown is Velpo Mabrey, who managed the Val Monte Shores resort for 11 years and Lake Guntersville State Park from 1970 to 1983. When he first moved to Guntersville after serving in World War II, he married local girl Sue Isbell. He served as president of the chamber of commerce, the Alabama Mountain Lakes Tourist Association, the Alabama Motel Association, and the Guntersville Civitan Club. (Lake Guntersville State Park.)

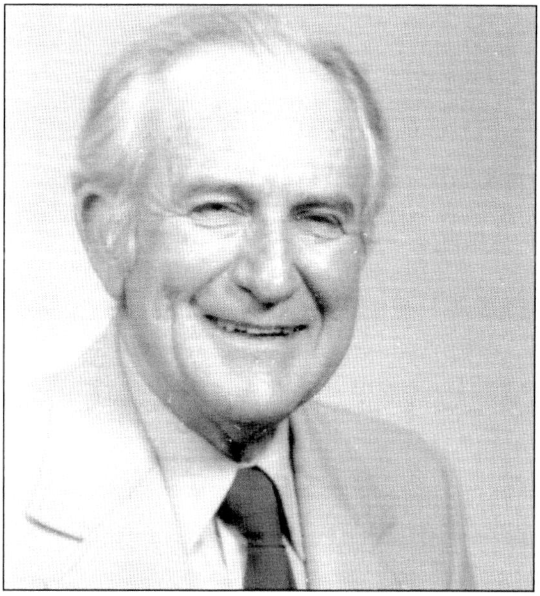

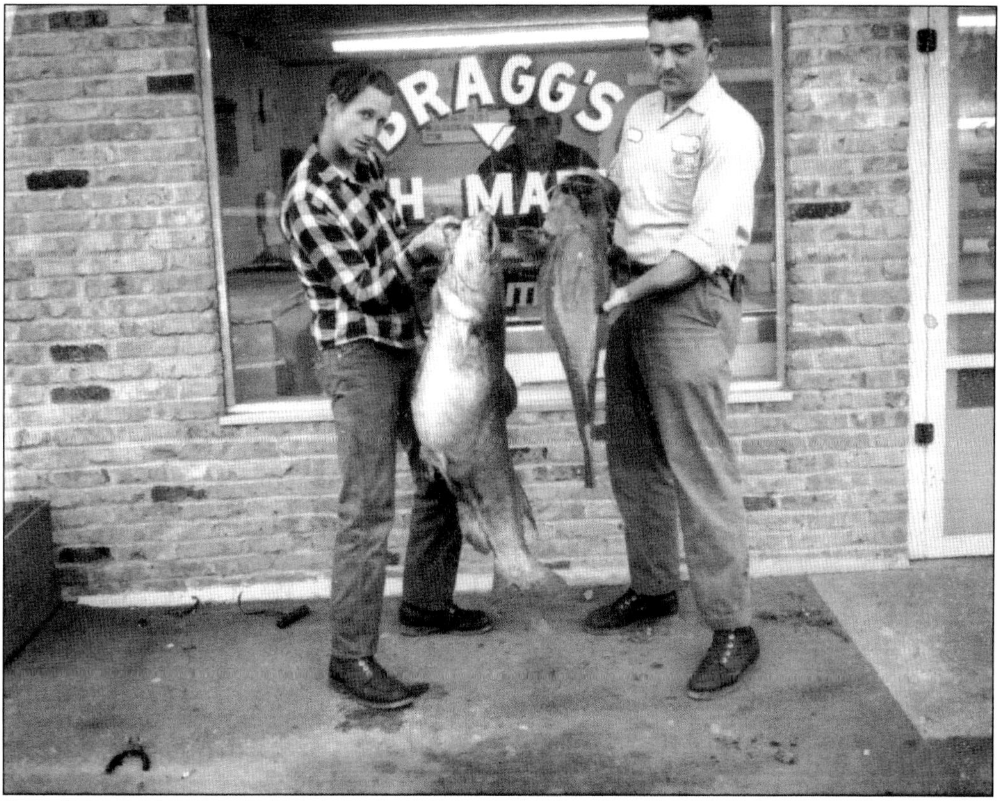

From left to right are Hewlett Moore, Leon Latino, and George Bragg. When Bragg's Fish Market opened in 1962, it gained its offerings from commercial fishermen. The son of a Birmingham fish market owner, Bragg loved fishing, hunting, and gardening. He served 12 years as president of the Guntersville Rescue Squad. He and his wife, Rose, had three children: Cheryl, Donna, and Mark. (Mark Bragg.)

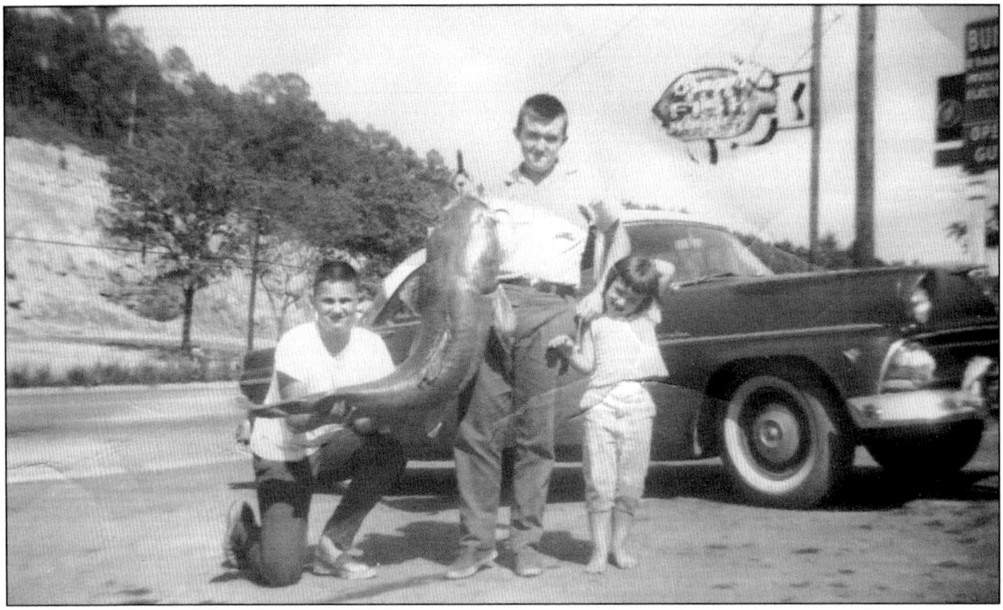

Pictured with this large catfish are, from left to right, Joey Breedwell, Curtis Bragg, and Cheryl Bragg. Fishermen with big catches often stopped by Bragg's Fish Market to take photographs. The original Bragg's Fish Market sign can be seen in the background. Today, the American Legion building is across the street. (Mark Bragg.)

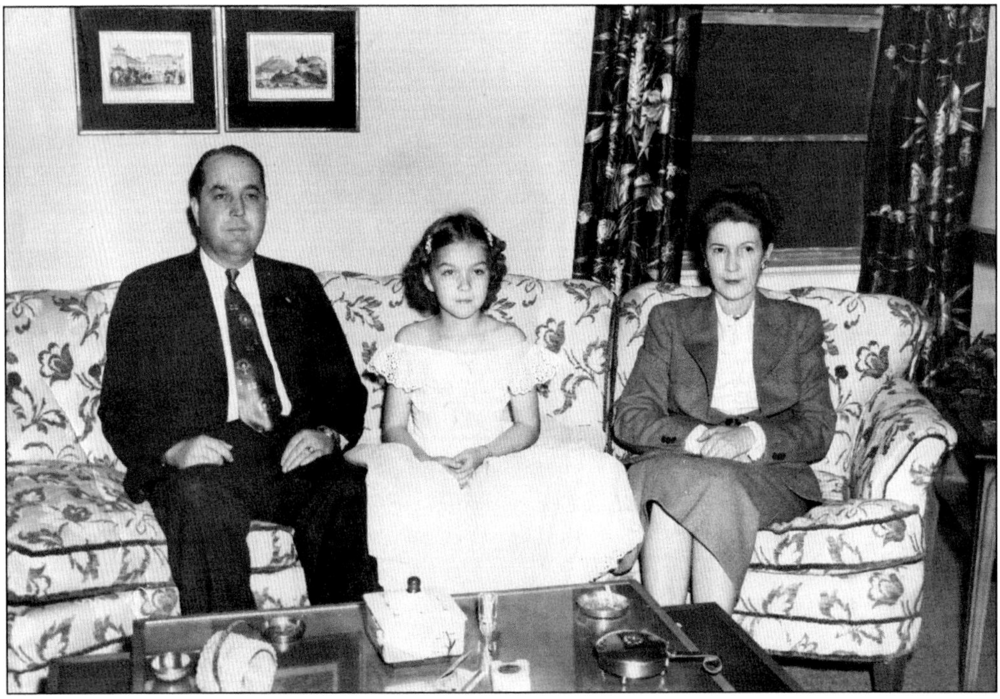

Taken in 1961, this photograph depicts T. Claud "T.C." Crain, his daughter "Little Elsie," and his wife, Elsie. He founded Crain Oil Company, a Shell distributor. Crain also owned a Buick dealership on Blount Street. It was purchased by Bob Hembree Sr. in 1956. Little Elsie married Sage Lyons Sr., who became state revenue chief under Gov. Fob James. (Marshall County Archives.)

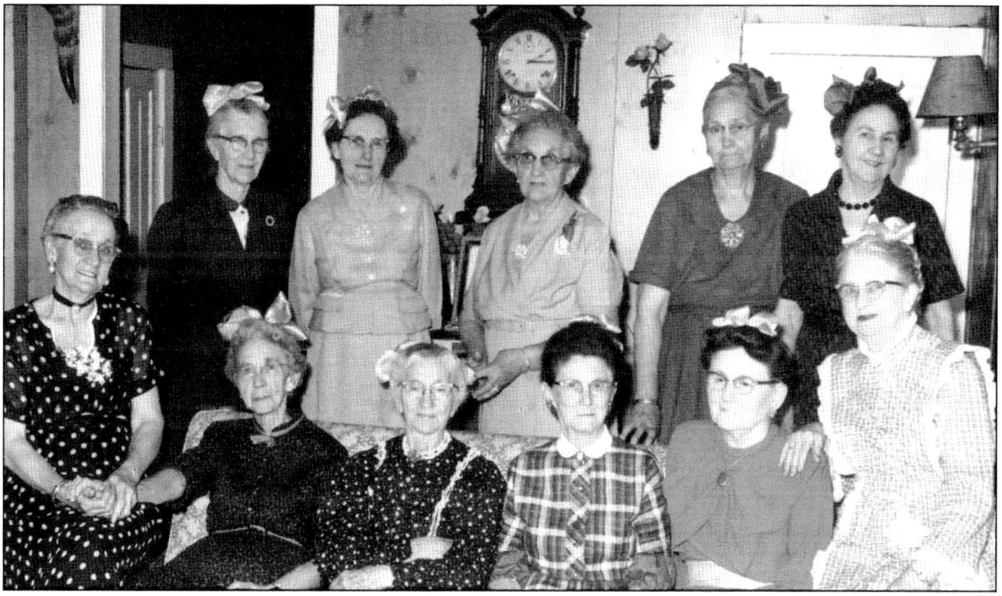

Having grown up at Diamond, near Guntersville, the "Diamond Girls" celebrated with activities like period costumes or the bows shown in this 1961 photograph. From left to right are (seated) Icel Smith, Frances Copeland, Lou McGee, Janette Moon, Margaret Taylor, and Hallie Whitlock; (standing) Suda Alldredge, Nova Jean Moon, Brunetta Coplin, Annie Claude Walls, and Dessa Pruett. (Marshall County Archives.)

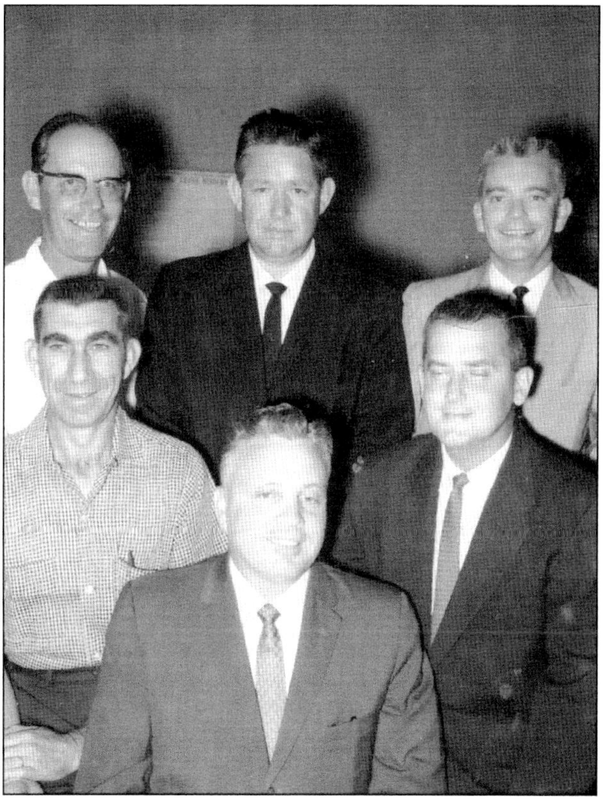

On June 29, 1961, these men were named Lions Club officers in Guntersville. From left to right are (first row) Pres. Aubrey Carr; (second row) Buel Locklear and Bud Abrahamsen; (third row) Robert McRee, Clayton Carter, and Bob Bishop Jr. (Marshall County Archives.)

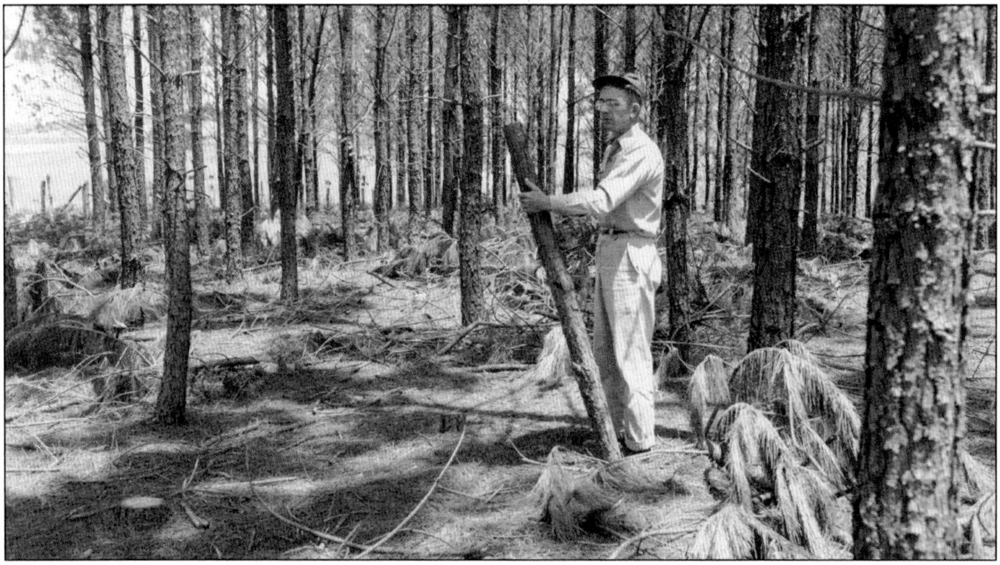

Kenneth Gross is shown harvesting a stand of pine trees for pulpwood on Georgia Mountain near Guntersville. As a farmer, he embraced crop diversification and grew cotton, corn, and popcorn. He used terracing and planted vetch to prevent erosion. In his youth, he worked for the Civilian Conservation Corps and the Tennessee Valley Authority. (Authors' collection.)

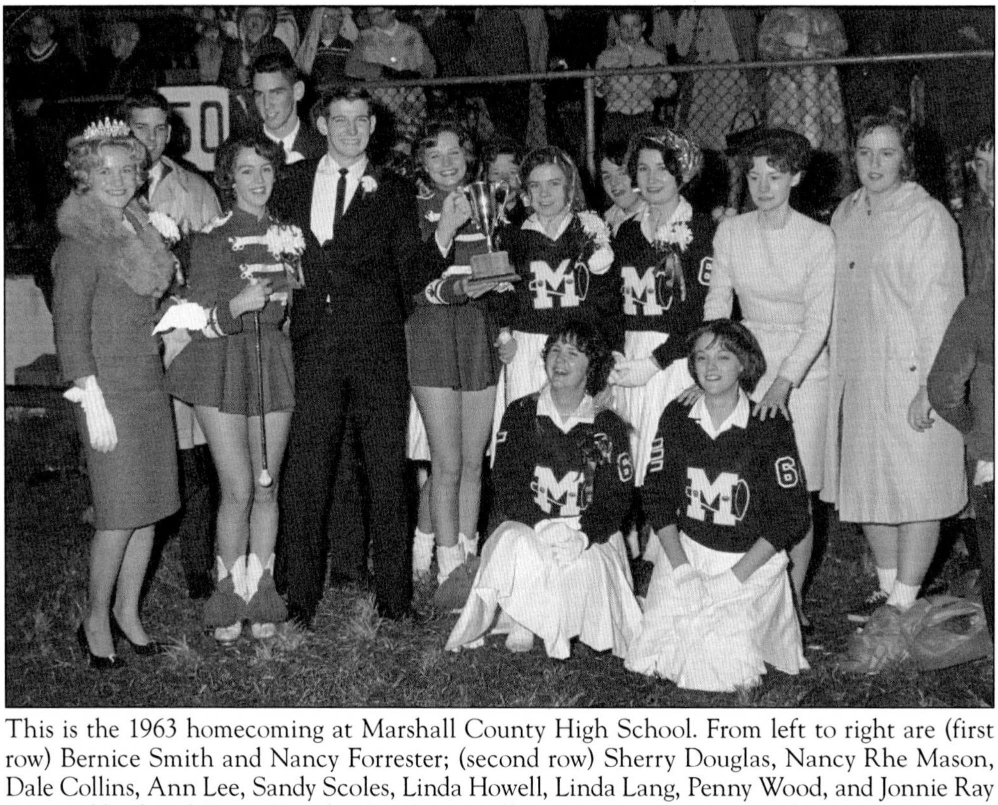

This is the 1963 homecoming at Marshall County High School. From left to right are (first row) Bernice Smith and Nancy Forrester; (second row) Sherry Douglas, Nancy Rhe Mason, Dale Collins, Ann Lee, Sandy Scoles, Linda Howell, Linda Lang, Penny Wood, and Jonnie Ray Baxter; (third row) Harry Douglas, Joe Scott Williams, Betty McGowin, and Karen Bosserman. (Authors' collection.)

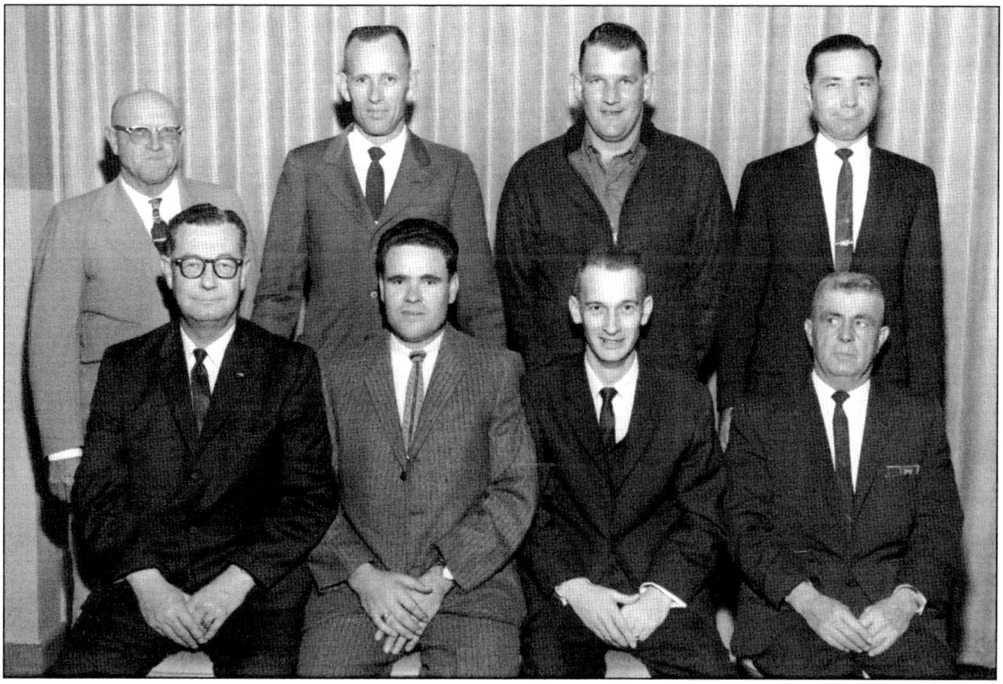

From left to right in this 1963 photograph are (first row) Sheriff L.P. Dickson, Chief Deputy Ralph Collins, Officer Deputy Buddy Albert, and Albertville deputy Wofford Chambers; (second row) jailer Troy Hughes and Field Deputies Troy Williams, Jimmy Weir, and Lowell Alewine. (Marshall County Archives.)

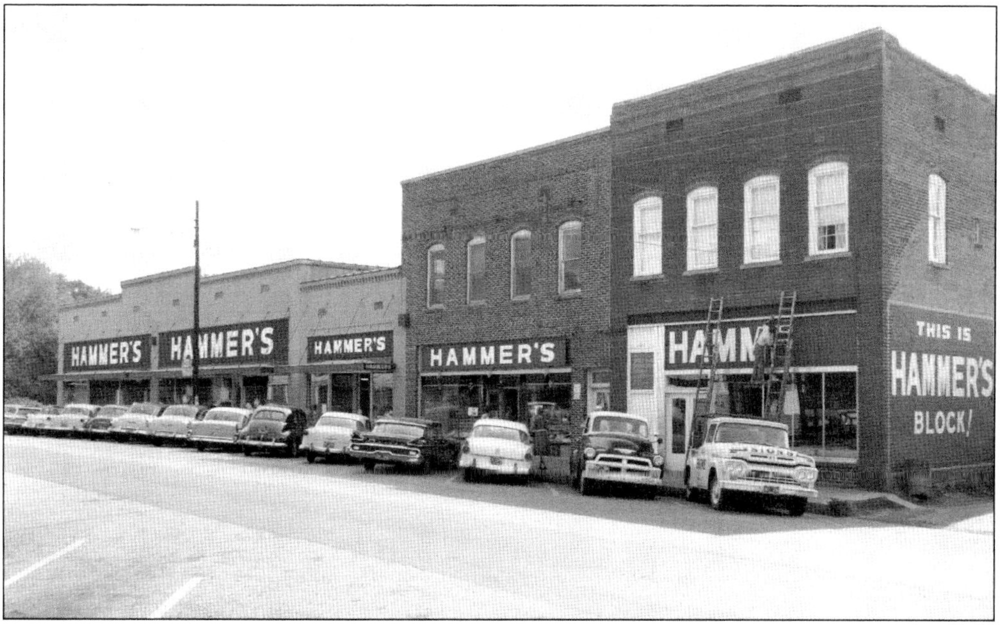

Located at the end of Gunter Avenue, Hammer's, now Fant's, offers discounted merchandise. Two of the five structures were built around 1907. Three of them have foundations with stone believed to be quarried locally. The city maintenance crews even discovered limestone curbs from the late 1800s. (Larry Smith.)

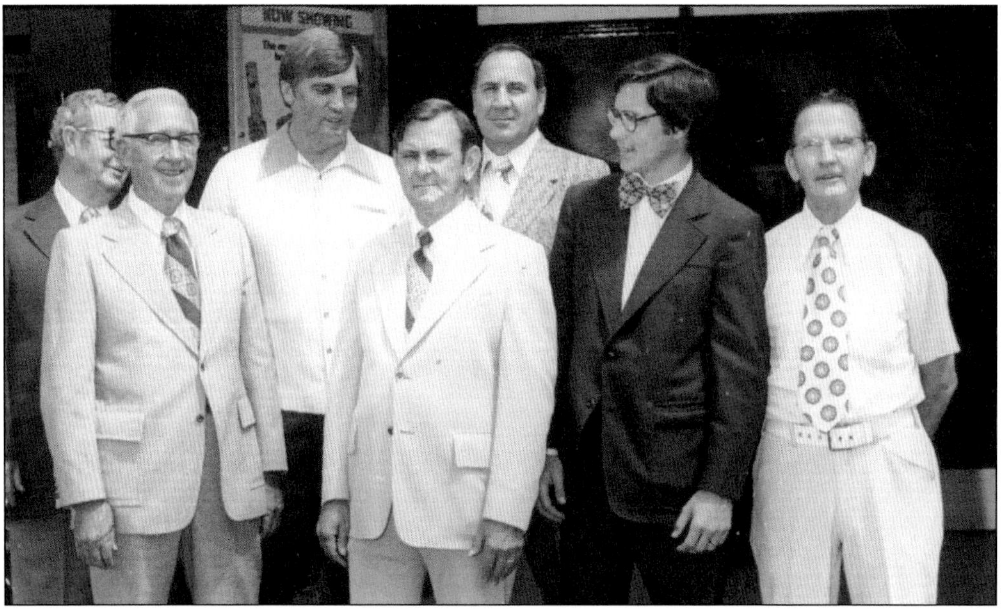

From left to right are L.P. Dickson, Buford Cryar, Buford Pusser, Billy Dyar, Rex Smalley, George Barnett, and Bill Harris. Pusser, the inspiration for the 1973 movie *Walking Tall*, made several appearances in Marshall County that year. He signed autographs at Guntersville's Lake Theatre, where the movie had a run of over two weeks. (Nancy Gilbreath Graham.)

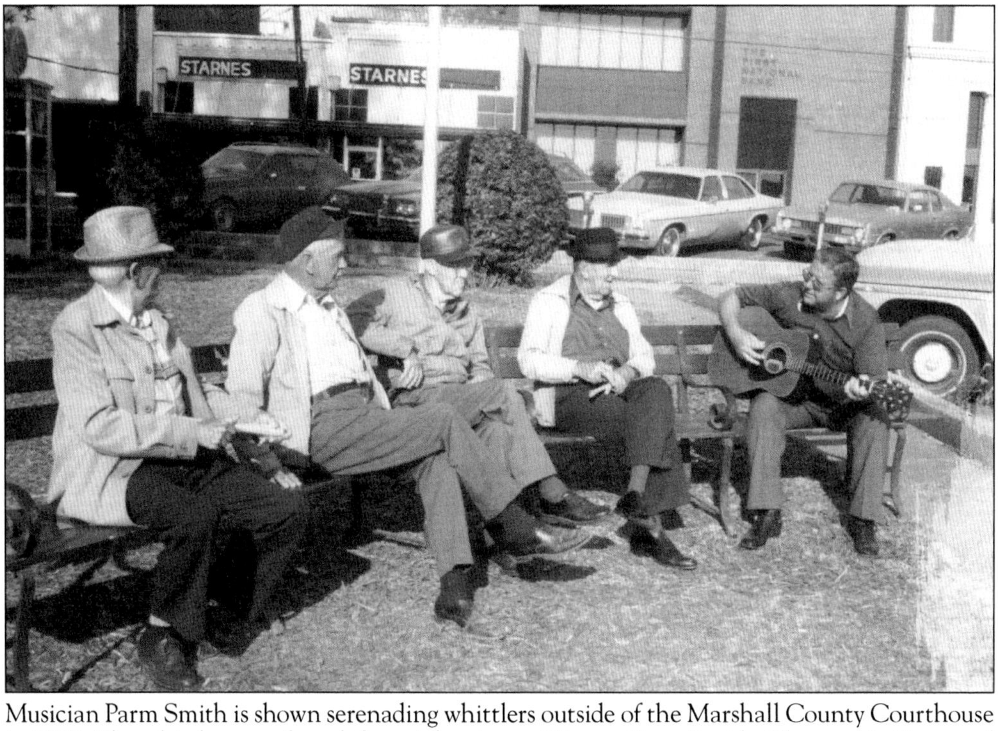

Musician Parm Smith is shown serenading whittlers outside of the Marshall County Courthouse in 1978. The whittlers are, from left to right, Amos Wisner, Drew Smith, Clarence LeCroy, and John Walker. According to the *Advertiser-Gleam*, Parm said the men should pay him to play, while the men replied "they would sooner pay him to quit." (*Advertiser-Gleam*.)

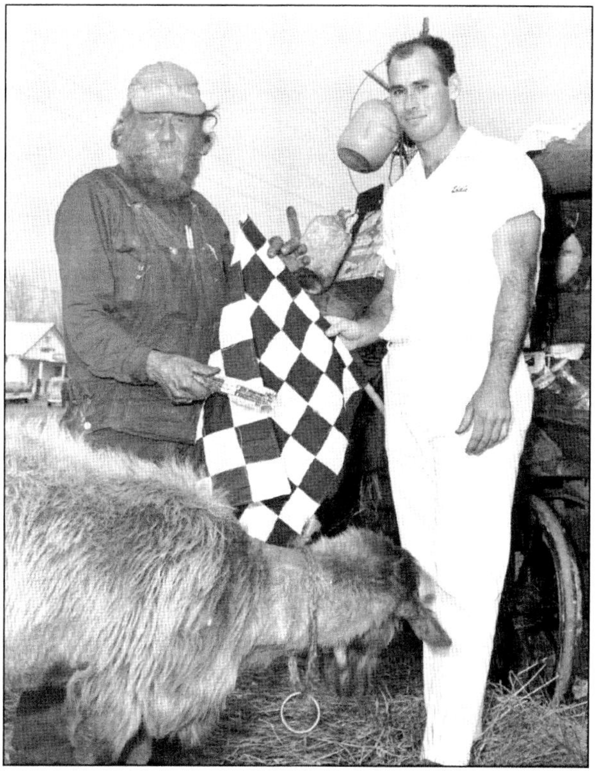

This is Charles "Ches" McCartney (left), the nationally known "Goat Man," and Eddie ? at the Gadsden Speedway. During one visit to Guntersville, McCartney claimed it had been 26 years since he had bathed. Of the goats, he said, "They don't care how I look or smell. They have faith in me, and that's more than I can say about a lot of people." (Etowah Historical Society.)

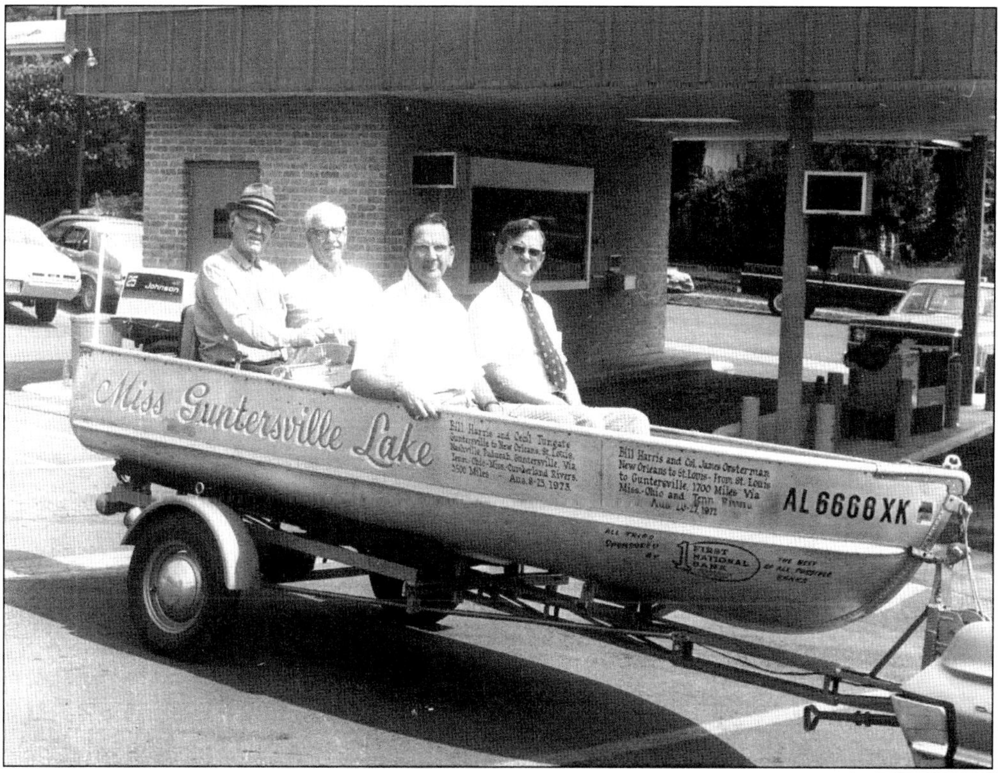

Sitting, from left to right, in the boat *Miss Guntersville Lake* are J.P. Willis Sr., Porter Harvey, Billy Dyar, and Bill Harris. The text on the side explains that in 1972, Harris and Cecil Tungate traveled 3,500 miles. It also mentions that in 1975, Harris and James Orsterman journeyed 1,700 miles. In total, Harris accumulated 55,000 miles with the boat. (Gail Smith Ingrum.)

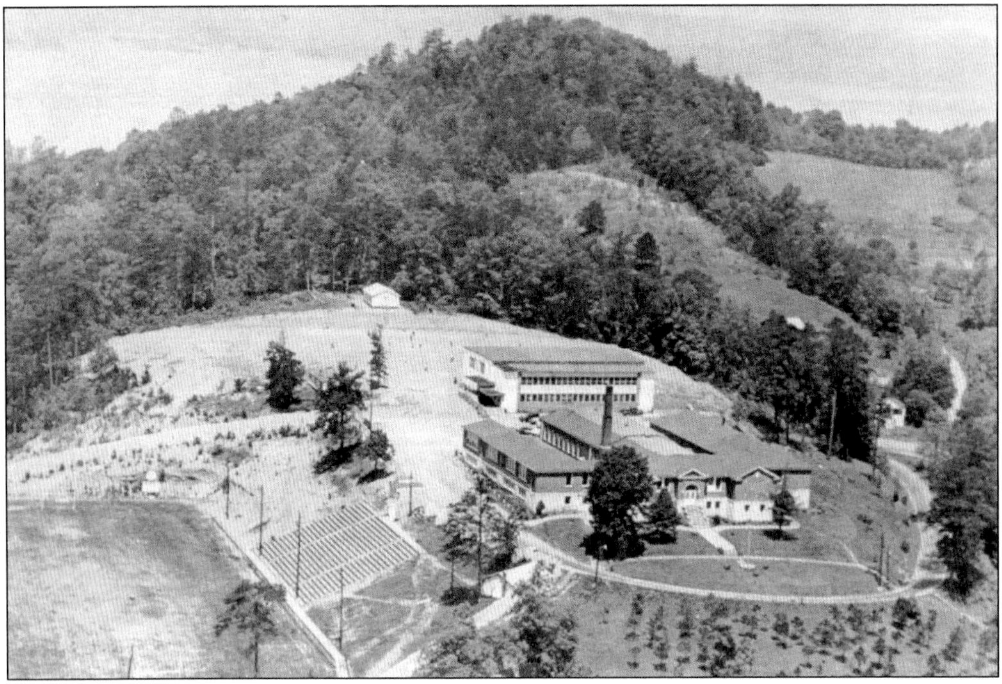

Marshall County High School, built in 1912, had a unique location "out on the hills of Marshall," according to the lyrics of the alma mater. Burned in 1930, the structure was rebuilt and used until 1971. Over time, the facility was enlarged with accoutrements like a stadium, gymnasium, auditorium, and vocational building. Guntersville High School opened in the fall of 1971 at its current location on US Highway 431. (Larry Smith.)

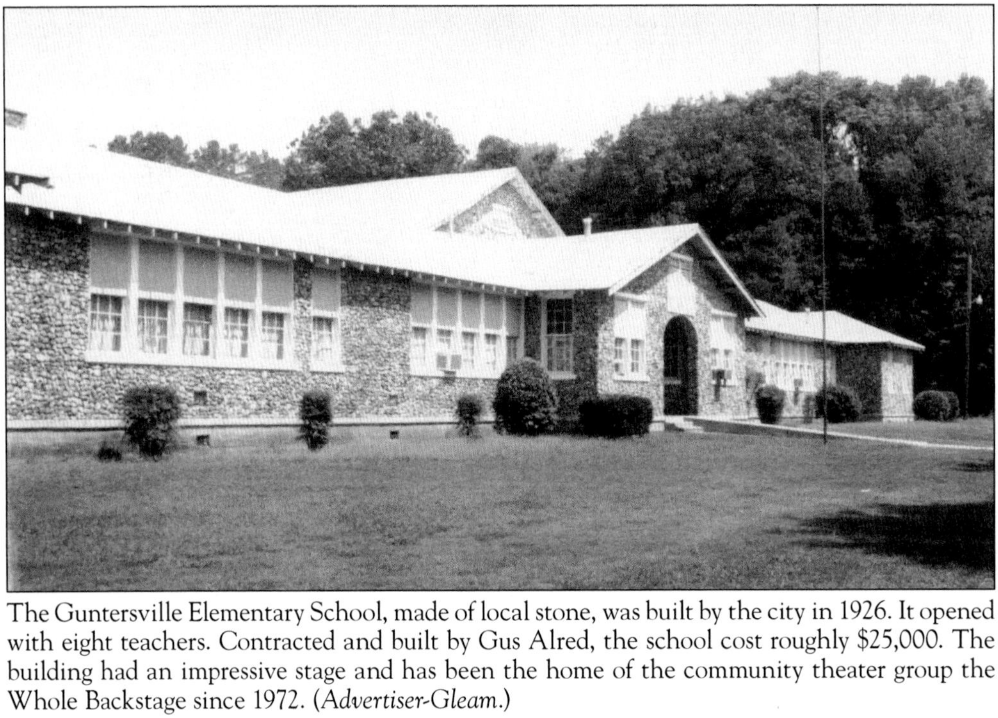

The Guntersville Elementary School, made of local stone, was built by the city in 1926. It opened with eight teachers. Contracted and built by Gus Alred, the school cost roughly $25,000. The building had an impressive stage and has been the home of the community theater group the Whole Backstage since 1972. (*Advertiser-Gleam*.)

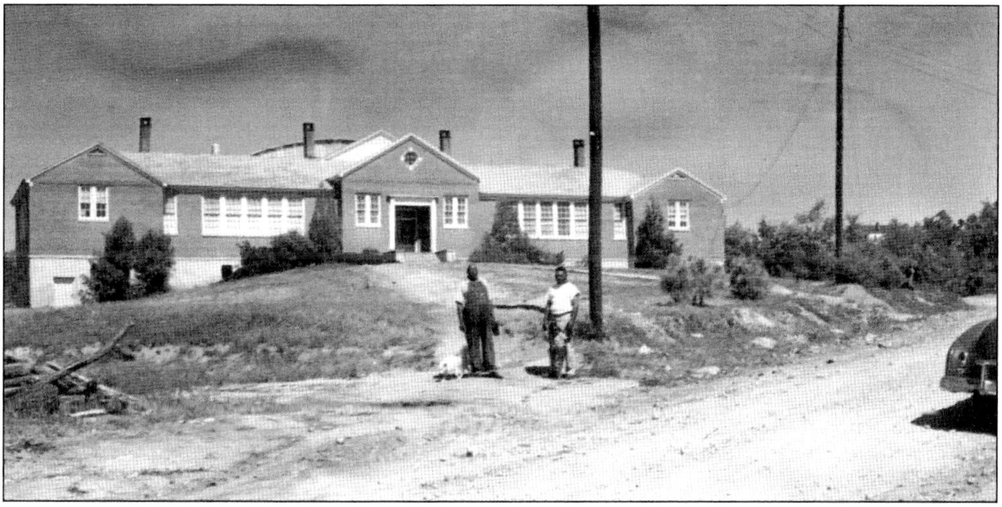

Opened in Guntersville in 1940, Lakeview School (shown above) offered black students the opportunity for education in Marshall County. The first graduating class was in 1942, and the last was in 1967. Enrollment declined when desegregation allowed transfers to other county and city schools. Destroyed by a fire in 1974, the building was replaced by a park named for longtime principal Roosevelt Williamson. (Larry Smith.)

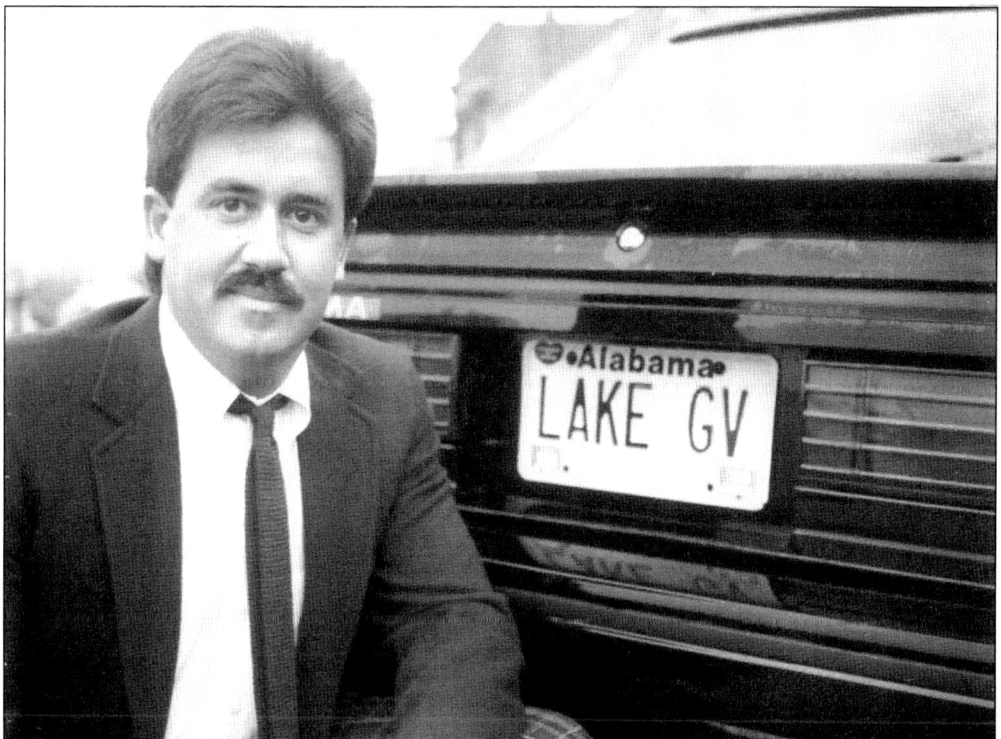

Walter "Bubba" Martin owns Bubba's II, a men's clothing store on Gunter Avenue. The son of Dick and Betty King Martin, he once served as president of the chamber of commerce and advocated changing the city's name to Lake Guntersville. He and his brother Rick have joked that they are the original "Rick and Bubba." (*Advertiser-Gleam*.)

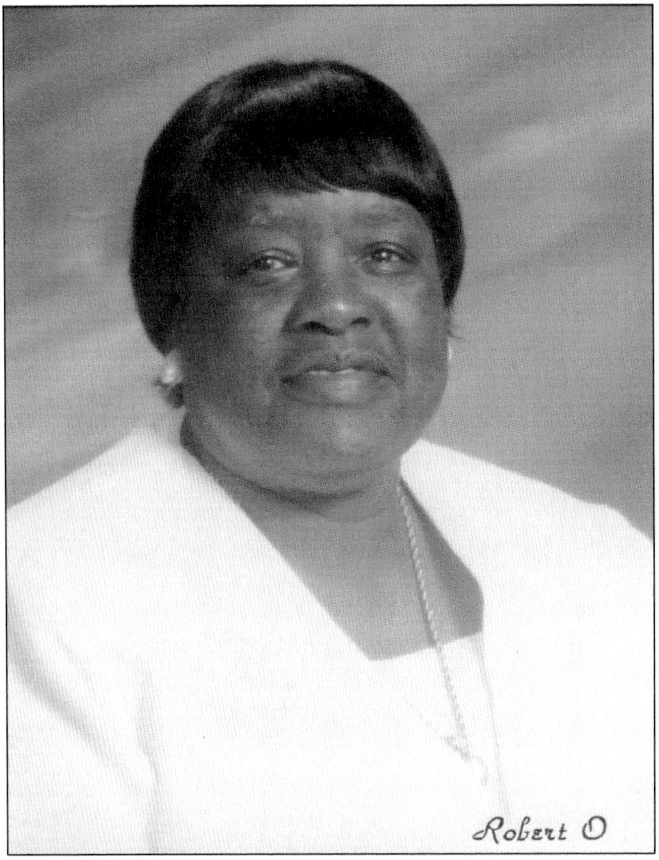

This is an undated photograph of former city councilwoman Nellie Franklin. The daughter of Addie and J.P. Sandridge, she graduated from Guntersville's Lakeview High School and from the Tuskegee Institute. She retired from the Bellefonte Nuclear Plant in Hollywood, Alabama. At one point, she served as matron at the sheriff's department. (*Advertiser-Gleam*.)

From left to right are Jerry Cornelius (booster club chair), Brandon Sparkman (superintendent), Percy Lee, and Joe Chorba. In 1987, the community named the stadium at Guntersville High School in honor of coaches Chorba and Lee. Their former players lauded them for teaching lessons in not only sports but also life. (Guntersville Historical Society.)

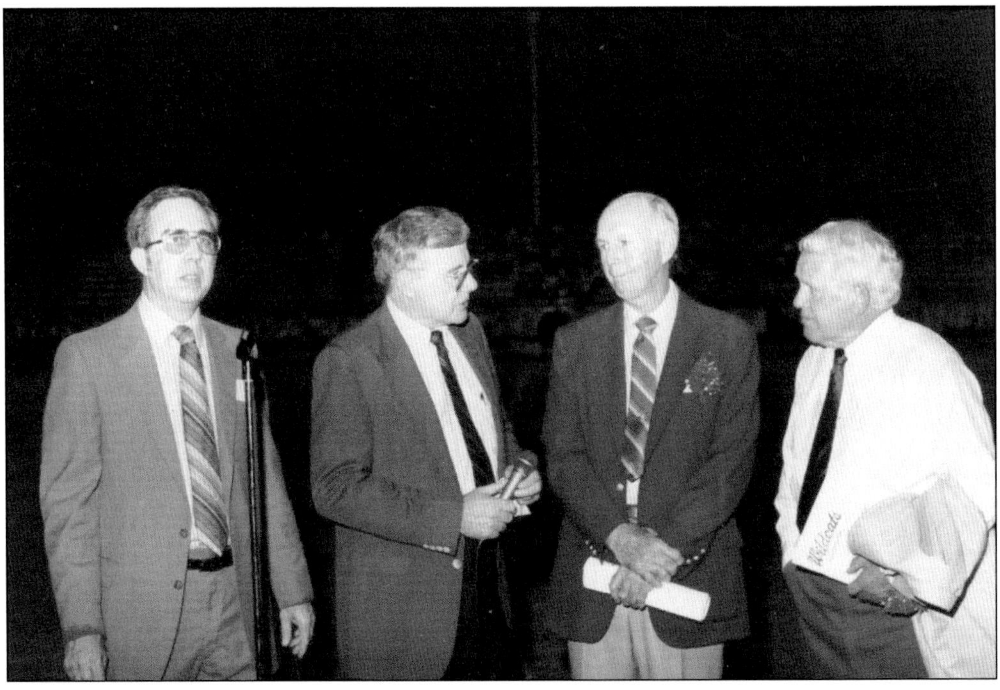

Louise Sahag (shown) was originally from Walker County but moved to Guntersville in the late 1950s and again in the 1970s, when she and her husband, Ed, lived at 608 Gunter Avenue. A charter member of the Ladies Civitan Club, she was also extremely active in the Marshall County Republican Party, regularly attended city council and city commission meetings, and ran for mayor in 1996. (*Advertiser-Gleam.*)

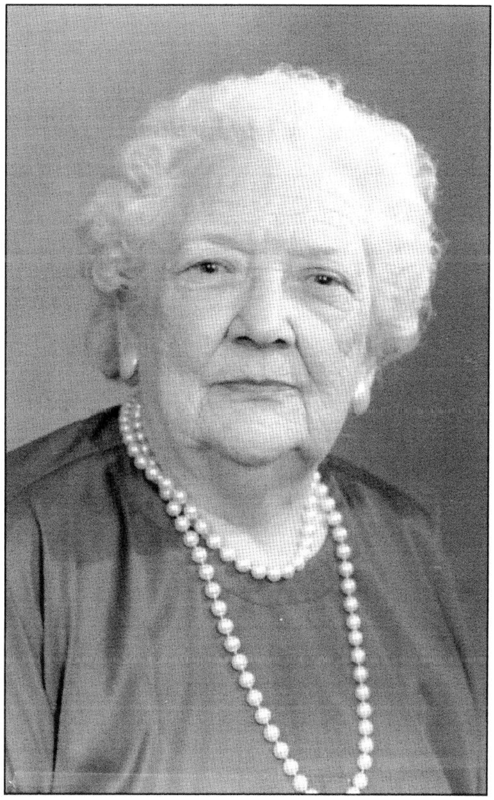

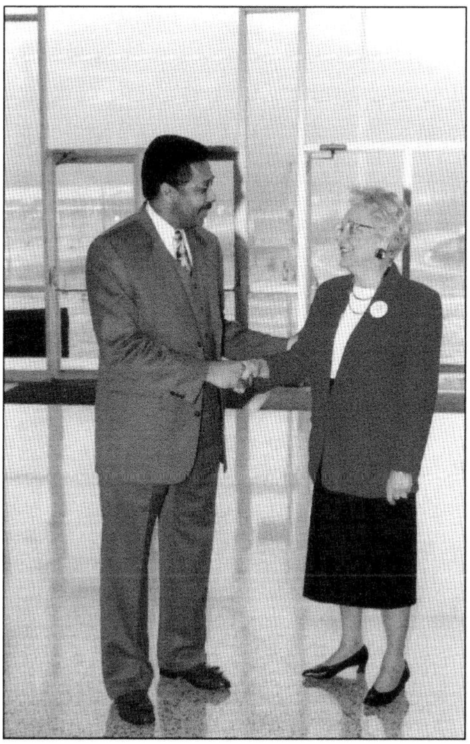

Johnny McAlpine, former president of Snead State Community College in Boaz, is shown with Annette Starnes. Starnes's membership in the Guntersville First Methodist Church spanned 80 years. She was heavily involved with the chamber of commerce as well as the Daughters of the American Revolution; Girl Scouts; Pilot Club; United Way; and Salvation Army. For some 30 years, she operated Starnes' Store. (*Advertiser-Gleam.*)

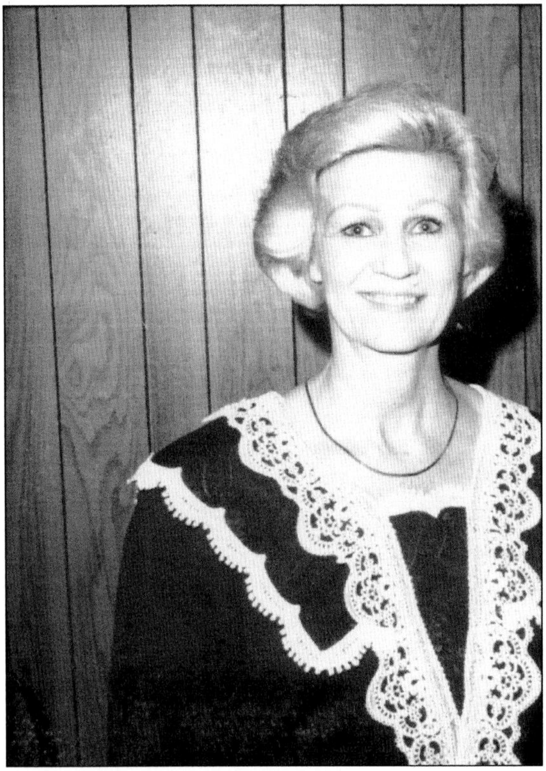

Jeannie Wallace (shown) served a long tenure as community education coordinator in which, among other things, she directed Marshall County Youth Leadership. She still keeps in touch with past participants in the program. Her civic involvement includes but is not limited to the Retired Senior Volunteer Program, Children's Policy Council, and Friends of the Library. (*Advertiser-Gleam.*)

Ed Neely (left) is displaying an image of a Union gunboat, while Grady LeCroy is holding a cannonball from the time Guntersville was shelled during the Civil War. When a young teenager, LeCroy found this cannonball in his yard at 337 Hill Avenue. In 1993, he donated it to the Guntersville Museum. (*Advertiser-Gleam.*)

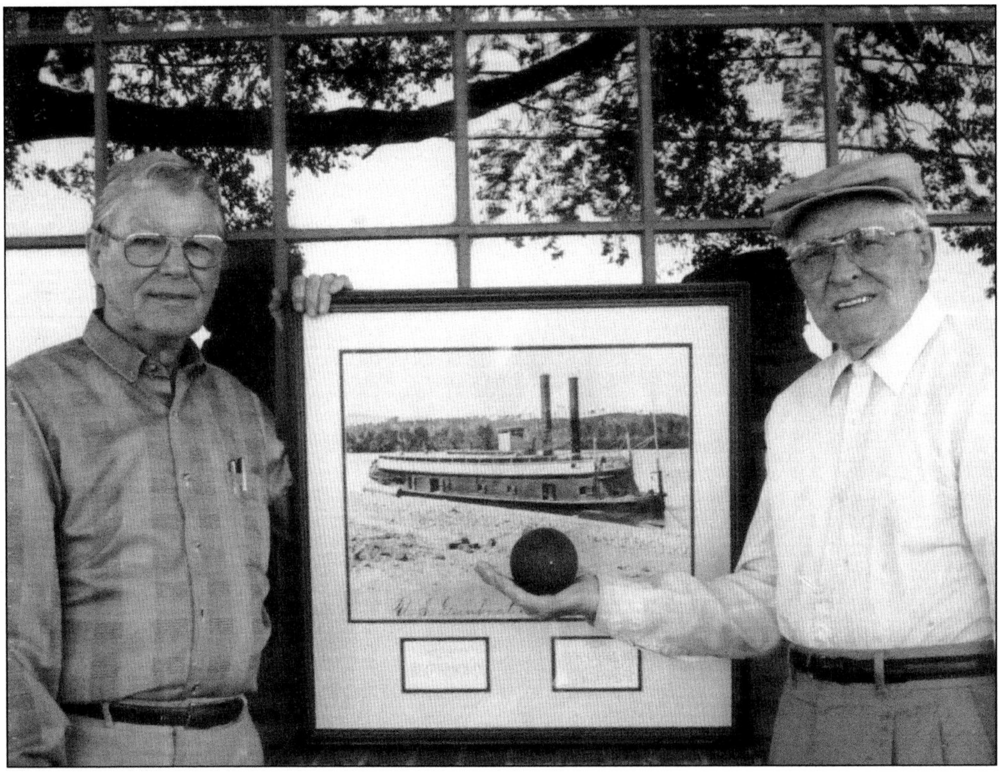

In 1980, Belinda Taylor became the first woman to serve as assistant county supervisor of the Farmers Home Administration in Marshall County. She earned a bachelor of science degree in agribusiness from Tuskegee Institute. She and her husband, Luther, had a son named Phineas Jamar. (*Advertiser-Gleam.*)

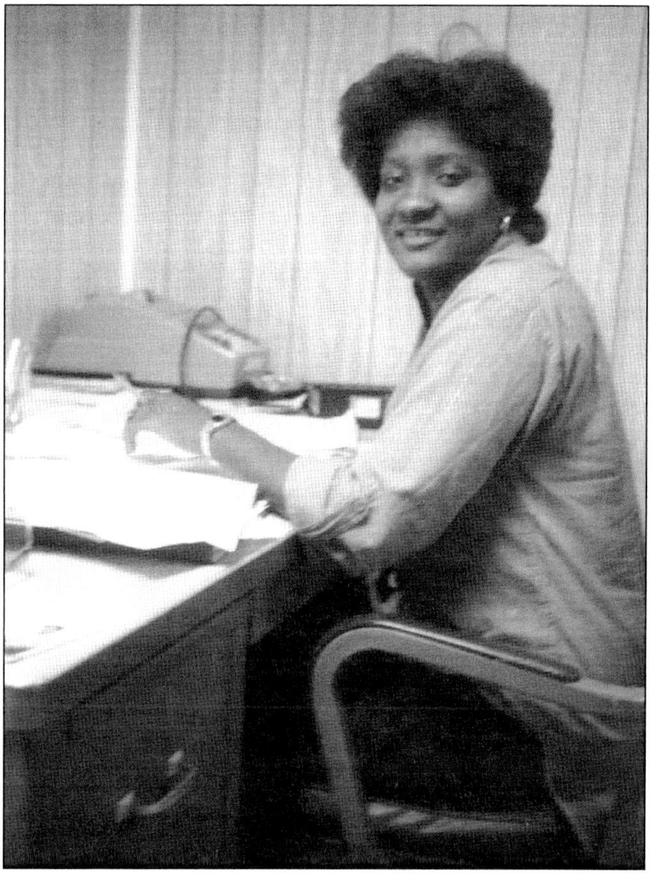

This postcard advertising Wanda's Restaurant and Ice Cream Parlor reads, in part, "near the courthouse, serving good food in a friendly, pleasant atmosphere. Also enjoy Sandra Clayton's paintings that adorn the walls. The customers are nice, too." The restaurant was owned by Jimmy and Wanda Selvage Poole. It was torn down in 2007, and the location is currently home to Errol Allan Park. (Nancy Gilbreath Graham.)

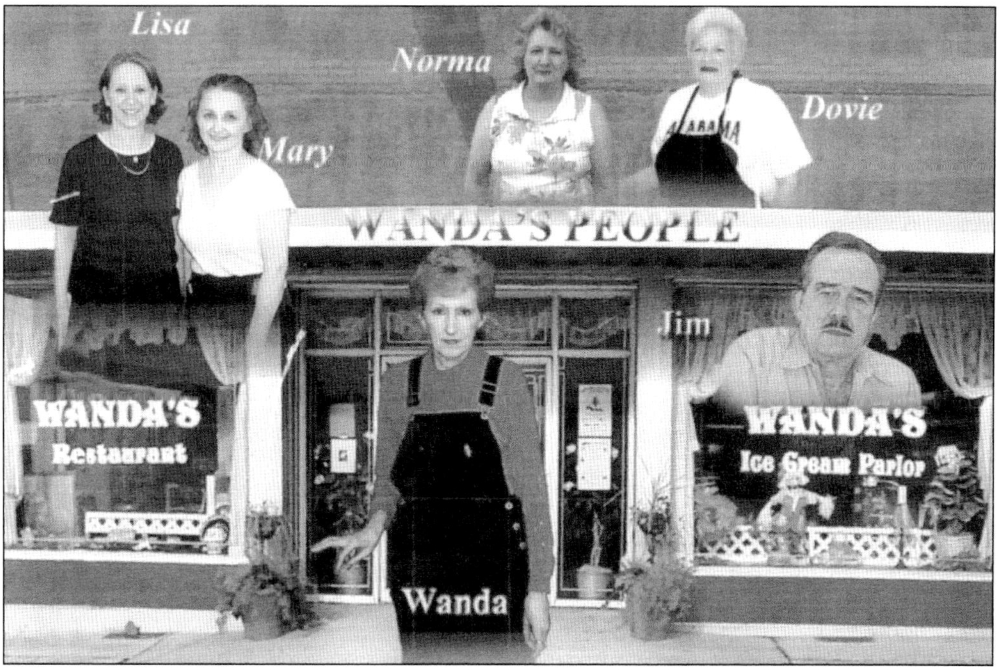

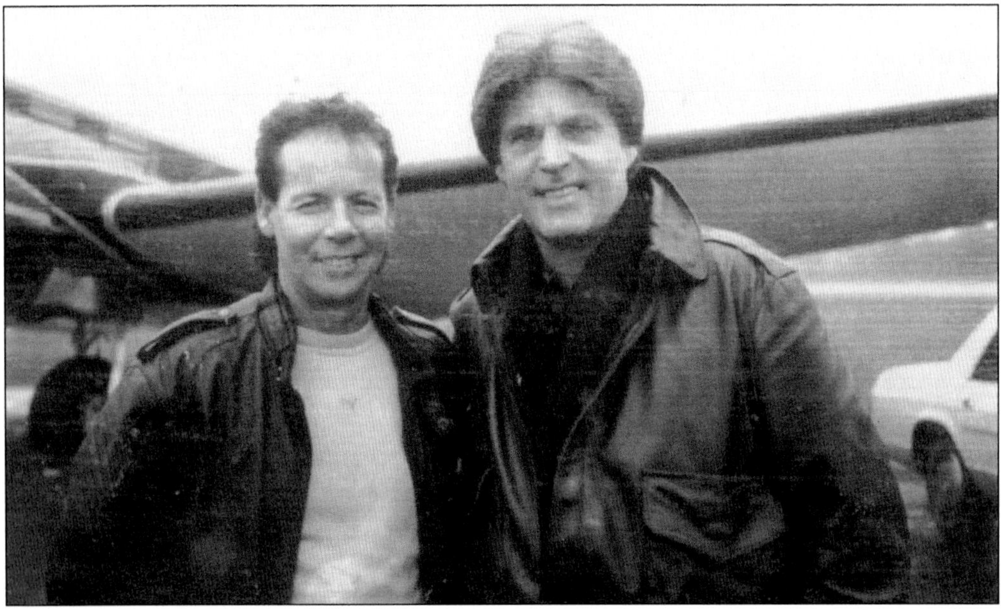

Pat Upton (left) and Ricky Nelson pose at the Guntersville Airport on December 31, 1985. Nelson performed two shows at PJ's Alley, a club owned by Upton, to roughly 500 people. Nelson performed favorites including "I'm Walking," "Poor Little Fool," and "Rave On." Traveling from Guntersville to Dallas that day, Nelson, his fiancée Helen Blair, and five members of his Stone Canyon Band died in a plane crash. (*Advertiser-Gleam.*)

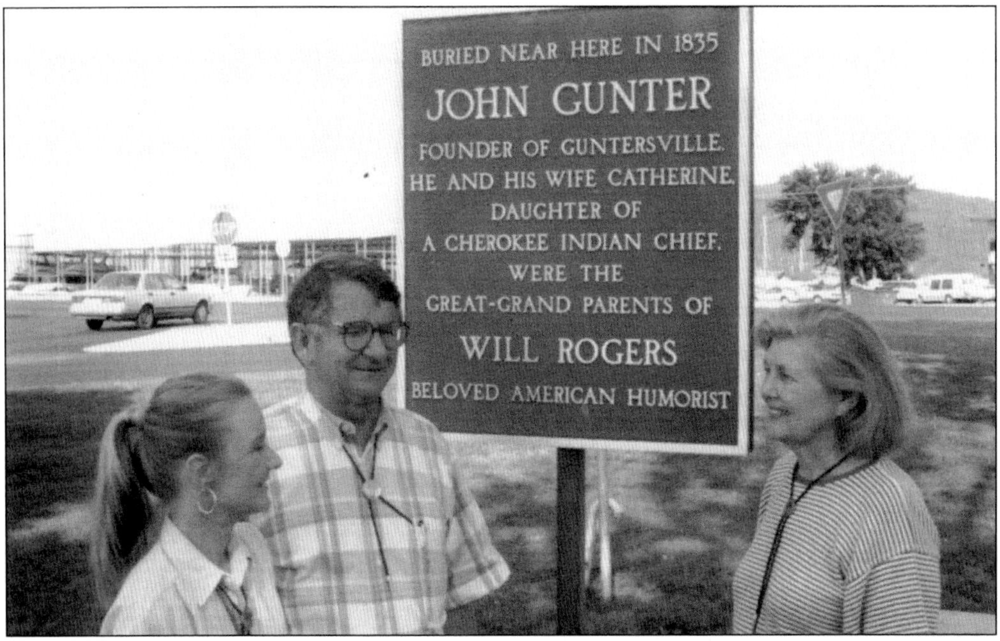
BURIED NEAR HERE IN 1835
JOHN GUNTER
FOUNDER OF GUNTERSVILLE.
HE AND HIS WIFE CATHERINE,
DAUGHTER OF
A CHEROKEE INDIAN CHIEF,
WERE THE
GREAT-GRAND PARENTS OF
WILL ROGERS
BELOVED AMERICAN HUMORIST

From left to right are Michelle Carter, Joe Carter (director of the Will Rogers Museum), and Ida Will Smith of the Guntersville Historical Society. Many in Guntersville embrace a tentative connection to actor, journalist, and folk hero Will Rogers, whose great-grandfather John Gunter founded the city. The Guntersville Museum has a life-size cardboard cutout of Rogers and a display about his ancestors and their importance to Guntersville's history. (*Advertiser-Gleam.*)

Elton Leon Kennamer was an internationally known photographer best remembered for working on location with natural light. Leon's Studio opened in Guntersville in 1955, after Kennamer's education in art at the University of Alabama and service in the Navy. He led seminars and conference in 39 states and seven countries. He married Bettie Scott, and they had two daughters, Milla and Lynn. (Milla Kennamer.)

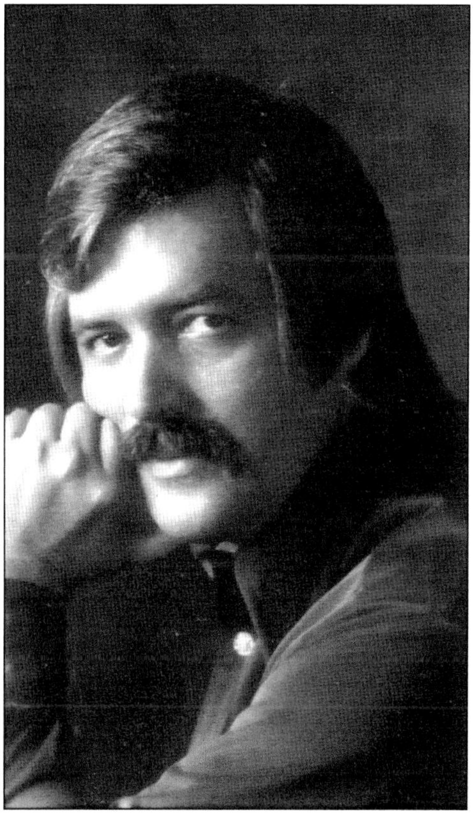

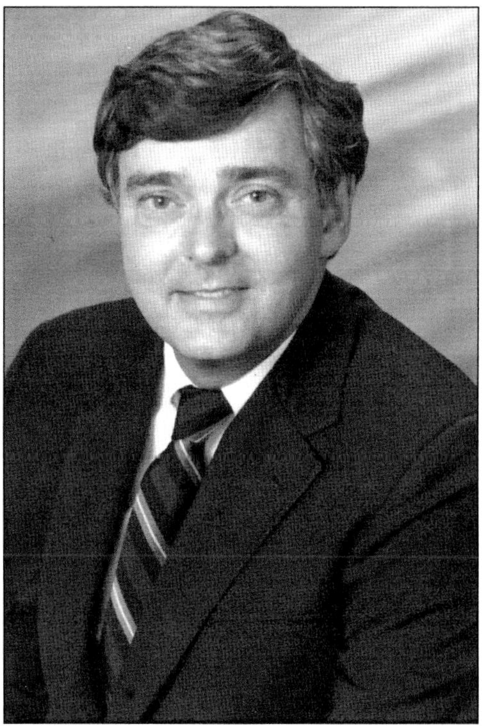

George Kappler, who previously worked for Monsanto, founded Kappler, Inc., in 1976. With his degrees in chemistry, he designed a line of protective clothing for use in medicine, industry, the military, and hazardous environments. Serving a global market, he employs 180 people and reflects proudly on his Alabama connection and the fact that his products are "Made in the USA." (*Advertiser-Gleam.*)

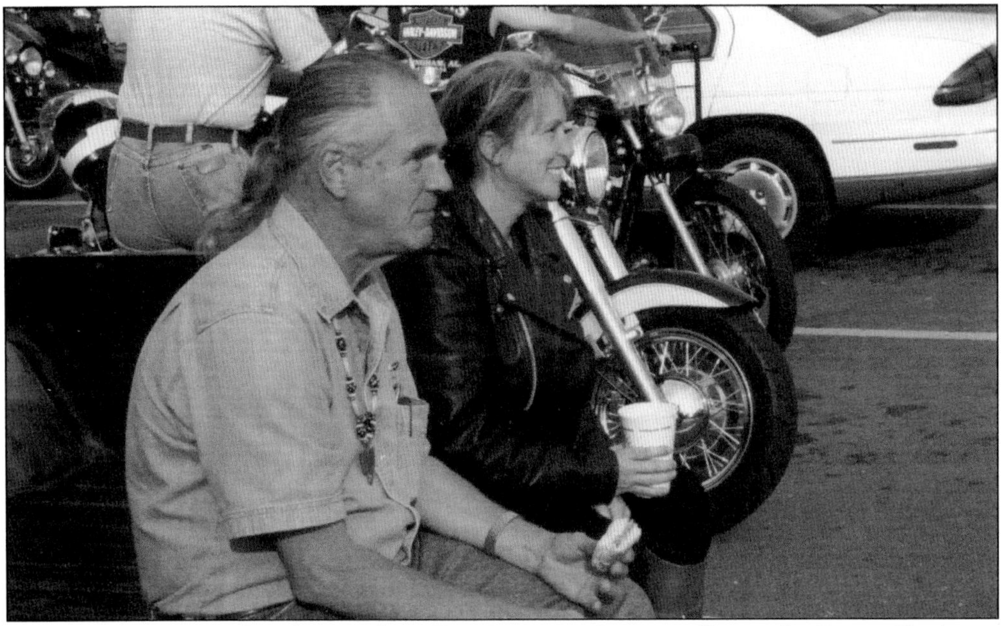

In September 2001, after driving from Fort Payne to Guntersville on the Benge Trail part of the Trail of Tears, Gina Still Waters Williamson and her husband, Leon Thunder Heart Williamson, are shown taking a break. Gina, who died in 2015, was chief of the United Cherokee Intertribal (UCI). In 2001, the Alabama Indian Affairs Commission recognized the UCI as a tribe. (*Advertiser-Gleam.*)

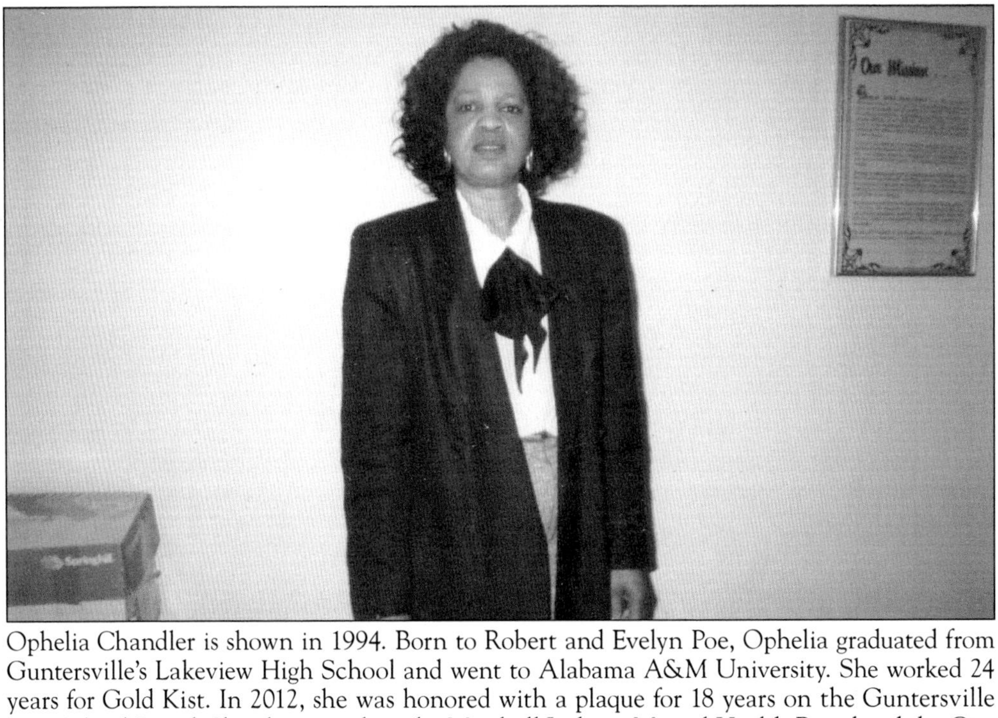

Ophelia Chandler is shown in 1994. Born to Robert and Evelyn Poe, Ophelia graduated from Guntersville's Lakeview High School and went to Alabama A&M University. She worked 24 years for Gold Kist. In 2012, she was honored with a plaque for 18 years on the Guntersville City School Board. She also served on the Marshall-Jackson Mental Health Board and the City Medical Clinic Board. (*Advertiser-Gleam.*)

Shown is Henry G. Lewis of Guntersville. He did not like the name Henry and preferred to be called "G." In 1900, he was born to John and Ada Lewis. He graduated from Marshall County High School, where he was a stellar quarterback. After attending Jacksonville College, he held a variety of jobs before becoming a salesman for Betsy Ross Bread and Meadow Gold Dairy. (Sonny Lewis.)

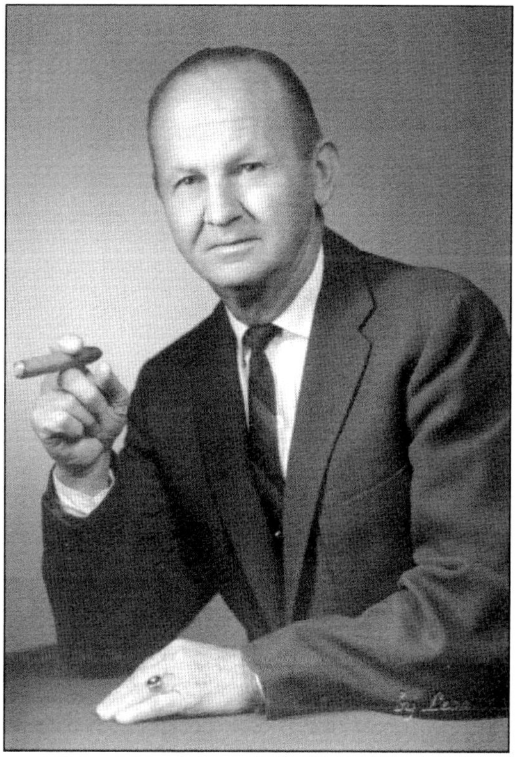

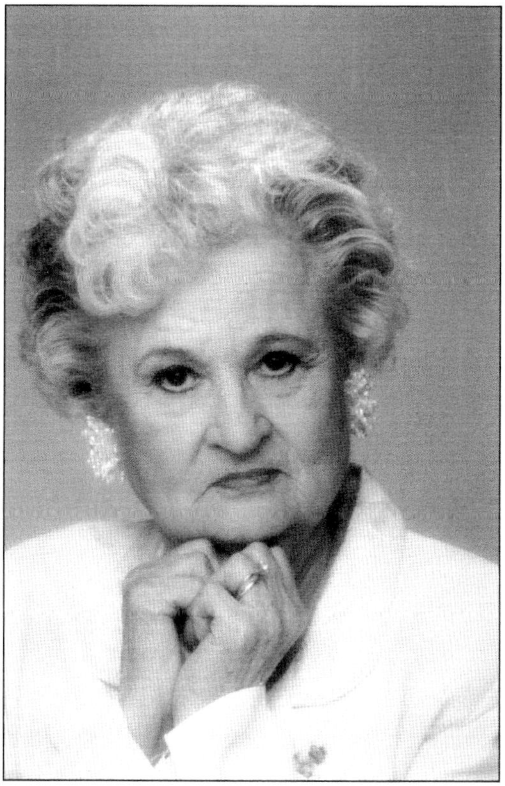

This is Margie Gilbreath Lewis Lane. She was born in 1918 in Guntersville, and her parents were Grover and D.C. King Gilbreath. In 1934, she married Henry G. Lewis. The following year, they had a son, William Edward "Sonny" Lewis. A gregarious lady, she managed a gift shop and spent over 22 years as manager for the medical clinic of Dr. John Boggus and Dr. Neal Christopher. (Sonny Lewis.)

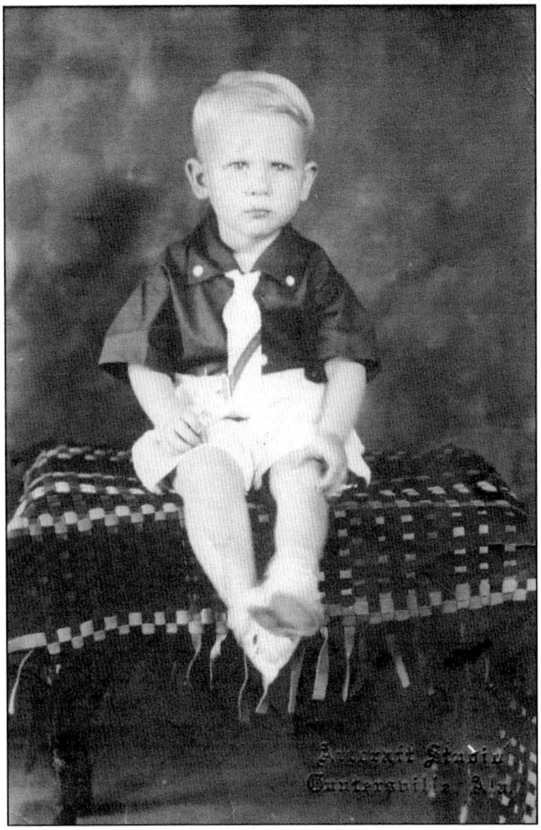

William Edward "Sonny" Lewis is pictured around 1940. He is a Guntersville philanthropist and local historian. He spent much of his life in California as a designer to the stars. The list of celebrities he met includes but is not limited to Doris Day, Diana Ross, Elvis Presley, and Barbra Streisand. He is affiliated with the Marshall County Archives, Guntersville Historical Society, and Guntersville Museum. (Sonny Lewis.)

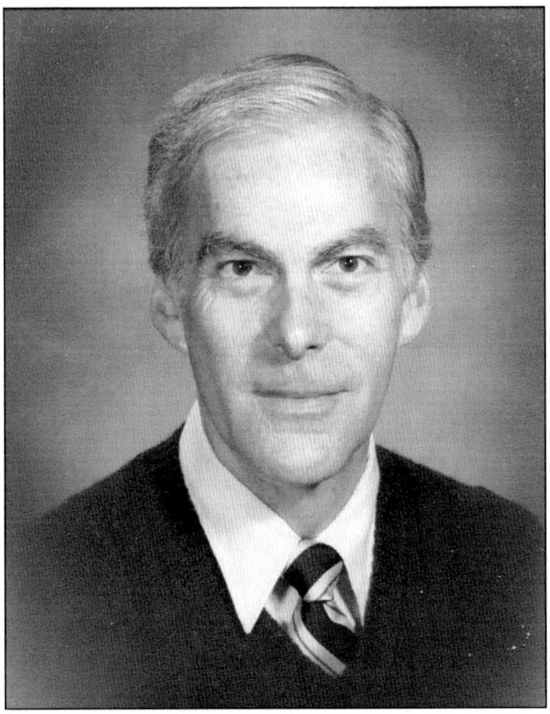

Errol Cross Allan, late Guntersville philanthropist and humanitarian, is the namesake of Errol Allan Park on Gunter Avenue. He donated $200,000 to the city so it could purchase the lot where Wanda's Restaurant was located. Allan was born in 1930 in Alhambra, California, and had a lengthy career as a high school teacher and counselor. He died in 2013. (Sonny Lewis.)

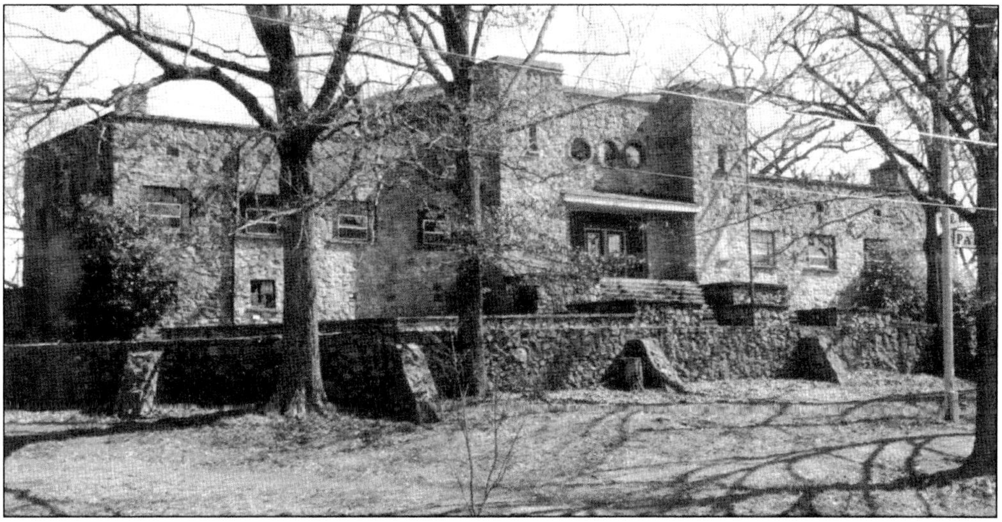

The Guntersville Museum and Cultural Center is at 1215 Rayburn Avenue. Among its diverse collections are displays on Native Americans, the Civil War, cotton, the Tennessee Valley Authority, veterans, and rocks and minerals. This building was formerly the Guntersville National Guard Armory, which, aside from contributing to the city's military history, also served as a social venue. (*Advertiser-Gleam*.)

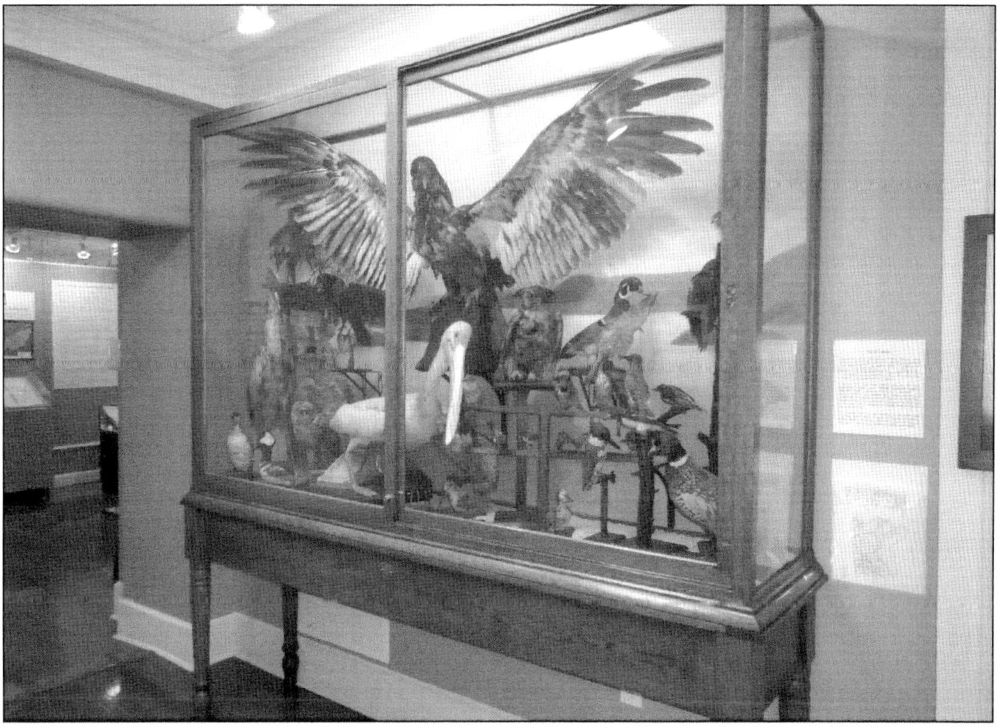

A self-taught taxidermist, Bessie Rayburn Samuel created this exhibit of 31 birds in the 1920s. For decades, the birds were in the front hall of the Guntersville Elementary School, but they are now displayed at the Guntersville Museum. "Bessie's Birds" continue to be admired by visitors of all ages. Some of the favorites in the display are the bald eagle, the great horned owl, and the yellowhammer. (Authors' collection.)

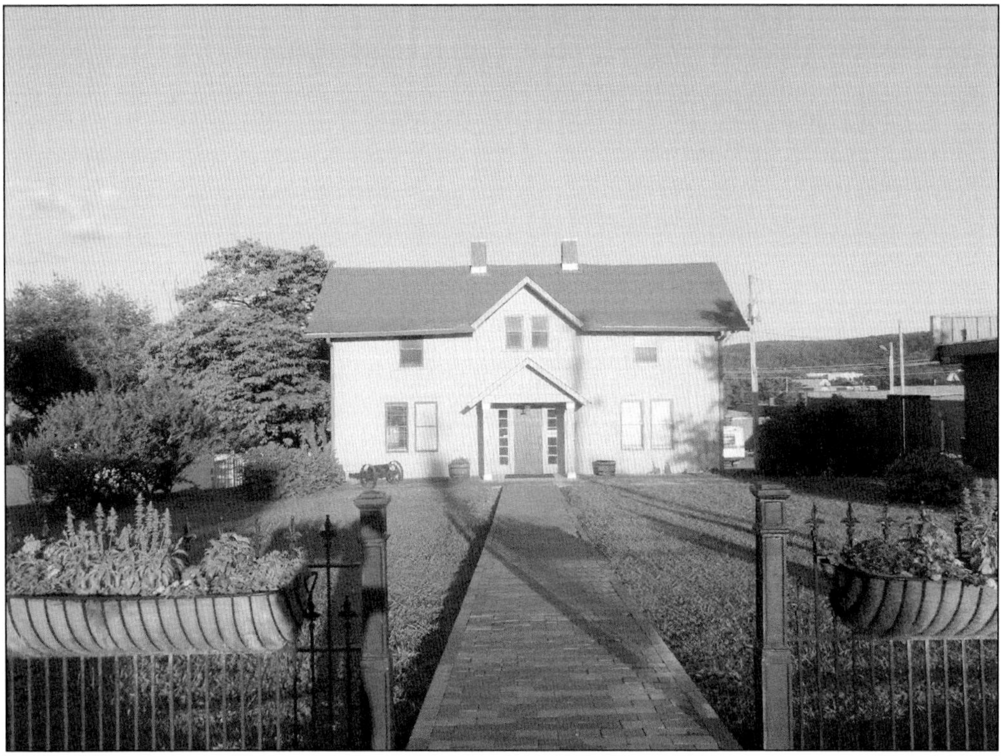

Located at 353 Blount Avenue, the Gilbreath House is the home of the Guntersville Historical Society (GHS). This museum has collections that emphasize Native American artifacts, an extensive Civil War exhibition, period furniture, and the creation of Lake Guntersville. In the summers, the GHS opens on Saturday from 10:00 a.m. to 2:00 p.m. for tours. The society also offers seasonal guided walking tours. (Authors' collection.)

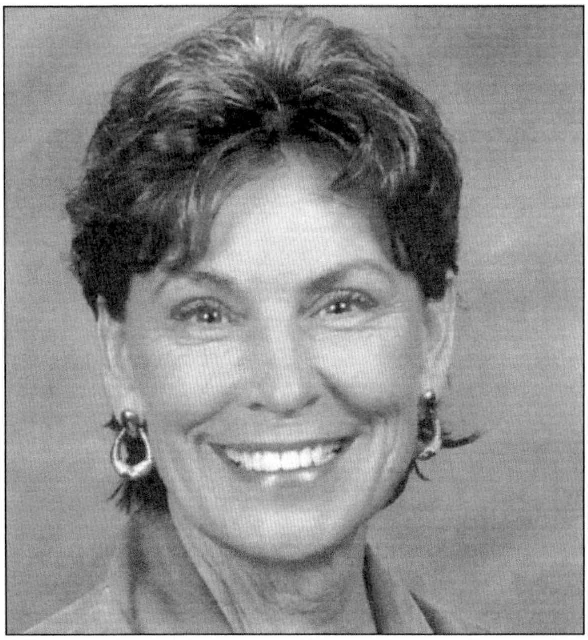

Macey Taylor is a local historian in Guntersville. Although she specializes in the history of buildings, especially houses, Taylor did pen an article that bemoans the loss of the old magnolia in front of city hall. A retired design consultant, she is a volunteer at the Marshall County Archives and is a member of the Guntersville Historical Society. (Marshall County Archives.)

Rosemary Roberts Darnell, an Illinois native, moved to Guntersville in 1976. She was among the first volunteers at the Marshall County Archives along with Betty Taylor and Margene Black. Rosemary and her husband, Lloyd, are the parents of two sons, Allan and Terry. (Rosemary Darnell.)

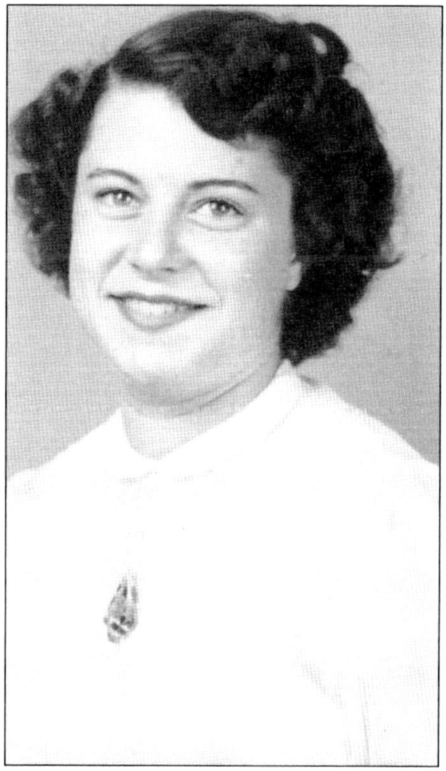

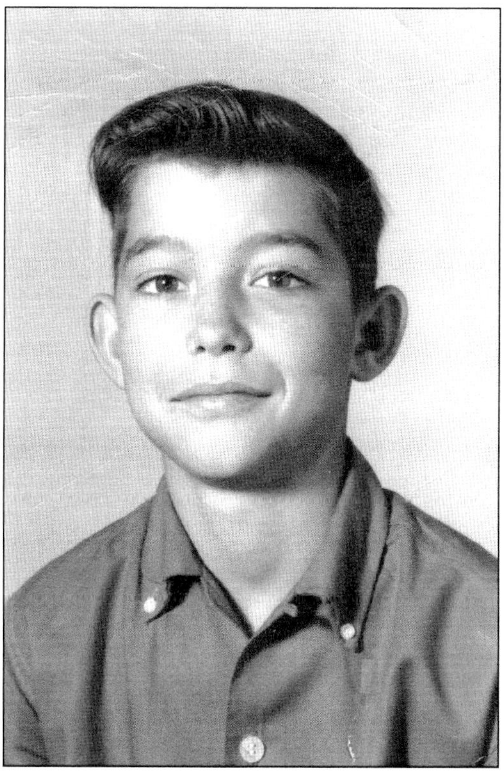

Having worked in computer technical support, Billy Alexander is an asset at the Marshall County Archives as its resident guru. His skills have resulted in many materials being posted online. Alexander, who has a wealth of stories to share, grew up in Marshall County but traveled extensively. This is his seventh-grade school photograph. (Billy Alexander.)

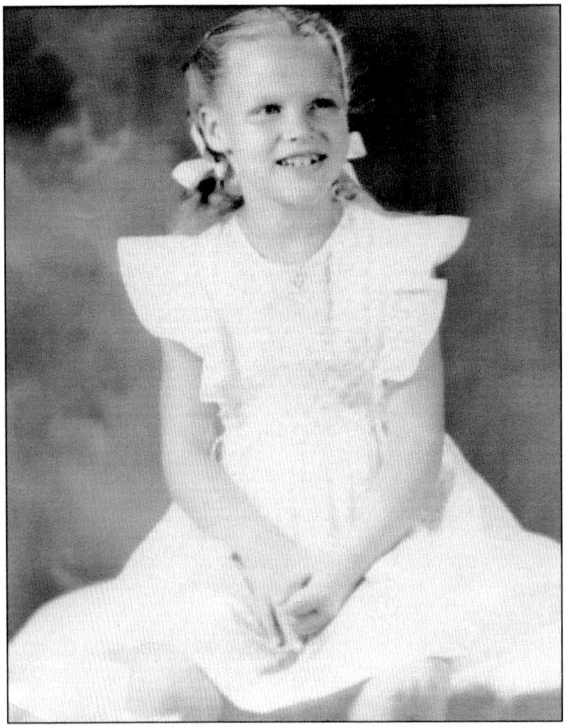

In this c. 1950 image is Margene Black, one of the earliest volunteers at the Marshall County Archives. She writes for *Valley Leaves*, the publication of the Tennessee Valley Genealogical Society. Some of the other early archive volunteers included Betty Taylor, Rosemary Darnell, Keith Finley, Lindy Hard, Rex Provence, Julia Rains, Martha Sharp, Neva Pascall, and Tempie Willoughby. (Margene Black.)

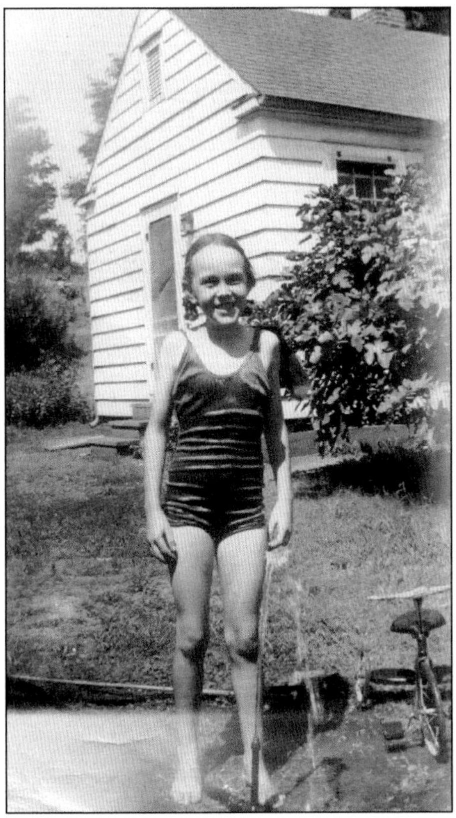

Betty Taylor, daughter of Quintus Donovan "Dono" and Loree Taylor of Guntersville, is pictured around 1941. In 1949, when 16, she was elected Harvest Carnival Queen. She is a retired schoolteacher and the current director of the Marshall County Archives. Her care and diligence has helped save many archival materials. (Betty Taylor.)

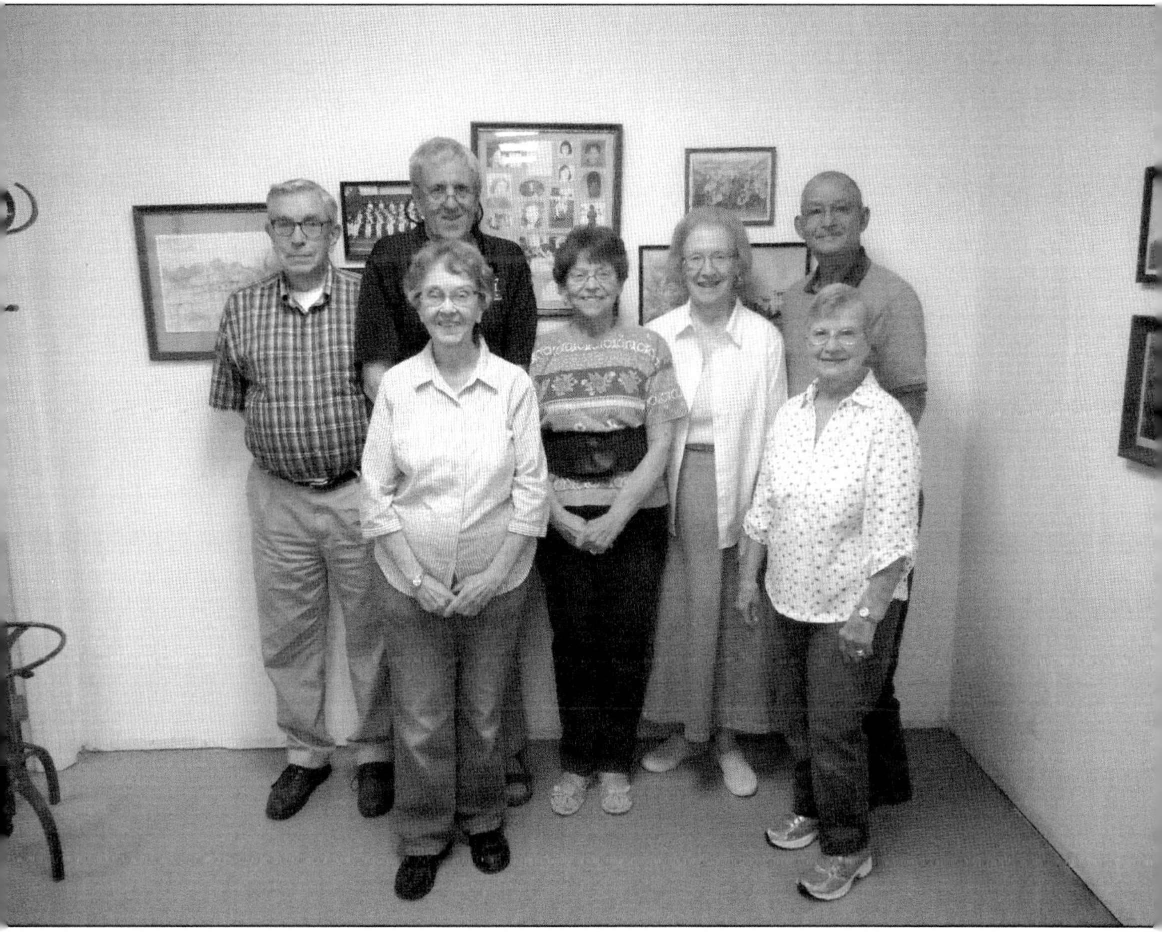

These are some of the volunteers at the Marshall County Archives in Guntersville. From left to right are (first row) Betty Taylor and Rosemary Darnell; (second row) Keith Finley, Larry Smith, Margene Black, Barbara Snow, and Billy Alexander. The archives began in the late 1980s, when volunteers were organizing documents in the Marshall County Courthouse for microfilm storage. In 1996, the archives moved to the Guntersville Museum, which at that time was in the old Episcopal church. The archives exhibited old pictures and family files. Around 2006, the archives moved to the corner of Worth Street and Blount Avenue. Among its holdings are bound newspapers, maps, photographs, marriage records, and family files. The Marshall County Archives is open every Monday from 8:30 a.m. to 1:30 p.m. (Authors' collection.)

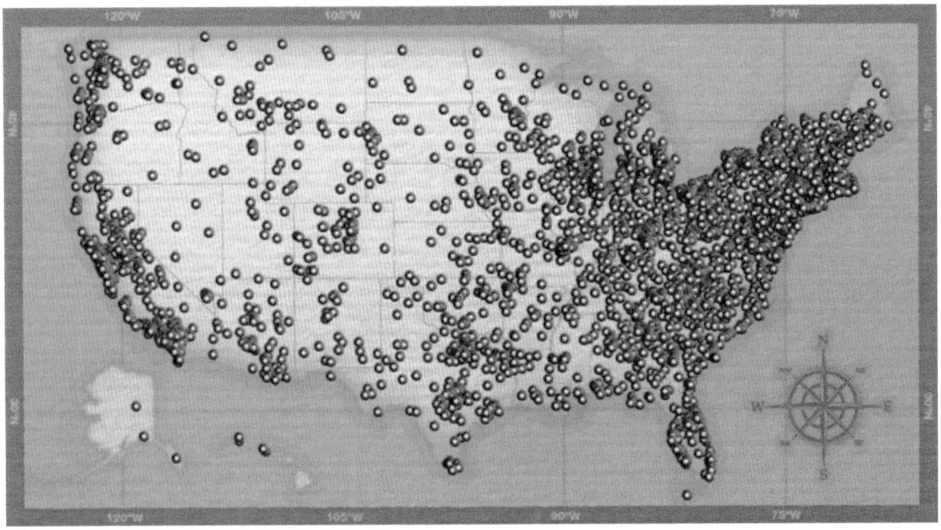